30-Day Anti-Inflammatory Challenge

A realistic approach to kickstart your anti-inflammatory lifestyle

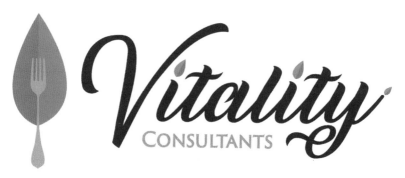

www.VitalityConsultantsLLC.com

ISBN 978-0-9910827-2-8

This book is for educational purposes. It is not intended nor implied to be a substitute for professional medical advice. The reader is encouraged to consult his or her healthcare provider before making any nutritional changes or following any nutritional program.

Printed in the USA

Table of Contents

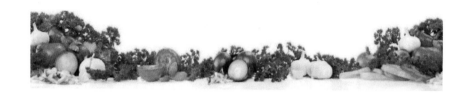

Why Did We Develop This Challenge?

If you have any experience with Feed Your Vitality, LLC you likely know something about our founder, Ashley Nanney. In 1998 Ashley was critically ill, overweight and hopeless. She knew that having a healthier lifestyle would make a huge difference in her health, but it seemed much easier to continue her current ways than to make any changes. Eventually Ashley was sent home with hospice and told by her doctors that she would die. This made something click with Ashley, and she decided she needed to make a change – not only for herself, but for her two-year-old daughter, Taylor.

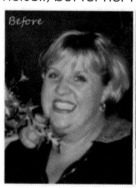
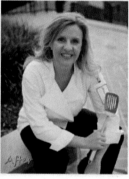

That is when Ashley began researching and becoming truly passionate about food, nutrition and wellness. She changed her diet and before she knew it, her whole life changed. Ashley is now 97 pounds lighter, no longer has health problems, and was able to watch Taylor, who is now 24, grow up. Ashley is a perfect example of how much a healthy can impact a person and is now dedicated to helping others change their lives

After years of cooking for and educating others about healthy living and meal preparation, Ashley decided to create this 30-day anti-inflammatory challenge to help others get a jump-start on their diet. This guide will walk you through the anti-inflammatory guidelines and give an explanation as to why some of the recommendations exist. Our hope is that this challenge will provide you with the framework you need to make an anti-inflammatory diet part of your life.

What is Inflammation?

Inflammation plays an important role in keeping the body healthy by protecting it from harmful bacteria, viruses and injury. Sometimes this inflammation goes overboard and attacks healthy tissue in the body. The way the human body reacts to inflammation is individual and can depend on genes, health status, diet, blood sugar regulation, stress and the environment. Inflammation causes the body to create free radicals, particles that can damage cells.[1]

Inflammation in the body can be acute or chronic. Acute inflammation happens immediately after tissues and cells are damaged and lasts for a short amount of time. Chronic inflammation lasts much longer than acute inflammation, up to several months or even years. This chronic inflammation can lead to chronic disease including arthritis, atherosclerosis, cancer, diabetes, hypertension, irritable bowel syndrome, lupus and multiple sclerosis. Factors that can lead to inflammation include smoking, stress, obesity, inactivity and diet.

If you have chronic inflammation in the body, you may experience one or more of the following signs and symptoms:

---

[1] Free radicals are by-products formed when oxygen leaves the cells. They are molecules missing an electron. As they pass cells in the body, they take electrons from them, leaving the cells damaged. Antioxidants are vitamins and minerals that can prevent and reverse damage done by free radicals. The largest sources of antioxidants are vitamins A, C and E, along with the mineral selenium.

- Aches and pains
- Congestion
- Diarrhea or irritable bowel symptoms
- Dry eyes
- Shortness of breath
- Fatigue
- Fever
- Frequent infections
- Indigestion
- Joint swelling
- Stiffness

The first step in reducing unnecessary inflammation is to keep the immune system healthy. What many people don't realize is that the digestive system plays a vital role in immune health. Eating the right type of proteins, fats and other nutrients can provide your body with the ingredients it needs to keep you healthy.

This challenge will walk you through the dietary recommendations for promoting immune health and reducing inflammation in the body.

What to Expect During the First 30 Days

After about a month, you will likely be adapted to an anti-inflammatory lifestyle and begin to experience some positive side effects. If you had symptoms from chronic inflammation prior to making these changes, they should slowly start to fade. You may notice that you have more energy, lost some weight, have fewer allergies and your skin is clearer.

Unfortunately, the first month of this diet may not be as pleasant as the side effects that occur after your body has adapted to the diet. If you currently follow a typical American diet, chances are that you are filling your body with chemicals and toxins. When your body gets comfortable with these toxins present, it goes through a withdrawal when you cut them out cold-turkey. When you stop consuming the toxins, your body will begin a detoxification. That is, it will start to clean itself of all the nasty chemicals that it has accumulated throughout your life.

When you read what your body is doing, it doesn't seem that bad. However, when you are experiencing it, you may feel like giving up on this lifestyle. Some people have cravings, excessive urination, fatigue, headaches, irritability and an increased appetite. If you experience any of these detoxification symptoms, you are likely wondering if the challenge is worth it. Let me tell you – it is! These symptoms usually will disappear from anywhere between a week and a month. When they do, you will begin to notice the awesome results that can come with an anti-inflammatory lifestyle. So whenever you feel those cravings coming, do yourself a favor: stay strong and say no! The longer you go without giving into those cravings, the sooner they will disappear altogether.

Along with the disappearance of cravings, you may also notice that you no longer get bloated. I'm not kidding. You're in the process of ridding your body of the "junk" that causes it to bloat. When you follow anti-inflammatory guidelines, you are not eating any of the foods that are associated with feeling bloated.

An added bonus to all of this is that if you are cooking for yourself, you will likely become much more skilled in the kitchen. You will learn to use ingredients that you may not have used before (coconut oil, almond meal, etc.) and prepare foods in ways that you are unfamiliar with (riced cauliflower, zucchini boats, etc.).

So remember, while they are unpleasant, side effects are likely to occur during this change. They are not permanent and should go away relatively quickly!

Allowable Foods List

FRUIT
Including but not limited to:

Apples	Lemon/lime
Apricots	Melon
Avocados	Oranges
Bananas	Peaches
Blackberries	Pears
Blueberries	Pineapple
Cherries	Raspberries
Cranberries	Strawberries
Dates/Figs	Watermelon
Grapefruit	Dried fruit
Grapes	(limited)

VEGGIES
ALL except white potatoes & corn

Artichokes	Mushrooms
Asparagus	Okra
Beets	Onions (all)
Broccoli	Parsnips
Brussels sprouts	Peppers (all)
Cabbage	Pumpkin
Cauliflower	Radish
Carrots	Seaweed
Celery	Snap peas
Cucumber	Spinach
Eggplant	Squash (all)
Greens (all)	Sweet
Green beans	potato
Kale	Turnips
Lettuce (all)	Zucchini

FATS & OILS
Clarified butter & ghee
Coconut oil/milk
Olive oil
Palm oil
Sesame oil (cold pressed)
Walnut oil (cold pressed)

NUTS & SEEDS
ALL except peanuts
Almonds
Brazil nuts
Macadamia
Pecans
Pine nuts
Pumpkin seeds
Sesame seeds
Sunflower seeds
Walnuts

LEAN MEAT, SEAFOOD & EGGS
Including but not limited to:
Anchovy
Beef
Chicken
Duck
Egg
Fish (all)
Lamb
Pork
Turkey
Veal

SEASONING/FLAVORING
Garlic/shallots
Ginger
Lemon/lime
Mustard
Natural herbs/spices (all)
Salsa (no sugar)
Vinegar

PANTRY ITEMS
Including but not limited to:
Unsweetened applesauce
Olives
Pickles
Pumpkin
Sun dried tomatoes
Tomatoes
Tomato sauce & paste

BEVERAGES
Almond milk
Coconut milk/water
Coffee
Green, white or herbal tea
Mineral water

TREATS & SWEETS
For occasional use
Carob powder
Dark chocolate
Honey
Maple syrup
Molasses
Palm sugar

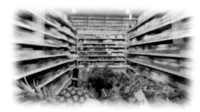

WHAT TO AVOID

Candy/junk	Overly salty foods
Corn	Processed foods
Dairy	Refined sugar
Inflammatory grains	Refined vegetable oils
Legumes	White potatoes
(including peanuts)	

Top 10 Anti-Inflammatory Foods

Almonds: Almonds are commonly referred to as a *superfood* because of all the great health benefits they provide. This type of nut has thiamin, riboflavin, biotin, folic acid, vitamin E, potassium, monounsaturated fat and protein. One serving of almonds, about one small handful, contains 40% of the recommended daily amount of vitamin E. This vitamin is an antioxidant that can prevent cell damage and boost immune health.

Blueberries: The deep blue color of blueberries is caused by a pigment with antioxidant properties called anthocyanin. This pigment protects the cells from inflammation and can increase the antioxidant effects of vitamin C. Blueberries also have fiber, manganese and vitamins C, E and K.

Broccoli: Broccoli is another food that is known as a *superfood*. This superfood has calcium, fiber, folate, iron and phytonutrients. One medium stalk of broccoli contains 12% of the recommended daily amount of fiber. Fiber can fight inflammation in the body by keeping your intestines healthy, regulating cholesterol levels and controlling blood sugar.

Brussels sprouts: Brussels sprouts are a vegetable that are

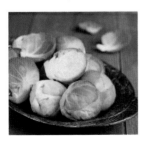 not included in many people's diet. However, they are packed full of anti-inflammatory and antioxidant nutrients, including vitamins A, B, C, E and K, calcium, copper, fiber, folate, iron, magnesium,

manganese, phosphorus, potassium and even protein. That's right, protein! One cup of Brussels sprouts contains 10% of the recommended daily amount of protein.

Flaxseed: Flaxseed contains many anti-inflammatory nutrients including vitamin B6, copper, folate, fiber, manganese and phosphorus. However, the largest of its anti-inflammatory properties comes from its high concentration of omega-3 fatty acids. These omega-3s protect the blood vessels from damage due to inflammation. Flaxseed has been shown to reduce C-reactive protein levels (a protein in the blood that measures inflammation in the body) by 10-15%.

Green tea: Green tea has many anti-inflammatory properties thanks to the large amounts of antioxidants it contains. Green tea has been studied for many years and may help control many inflammatory diseases including atherosclerosis, arthritis, diabetes, high cholesterol and inflammatory bowel disease.

Herbs and spices: Herbs and spices are an easy way to add anti-inflammatory properties to any meal. Our two favorites include ginger and turmeric. Ginger inhibits inflammatory enzymes in the body. It has also been shown to reduce pain caused by arthritis and increase blood circulation. Turmeric is the main ingredient in curry and has many anti-inflammatory and antioxidant properties. It works the same way as ginger by inhibiting inflammatory enzymes and can relieve indigestion, reduce pain caused by arthritis and improve circulation.

Mushrooms: Mushrooms may be one of the best food choices when it comes to fighting inflammation. Mushrooms contain many nutrients and antioxidants. In fact, a half-cup serving provides you with 50% of the recommended daily amount of the antioxidant selenium. Mushrooms have been shown to help white blood cells protect the body against infection, heart disease, cancer and arthritis.

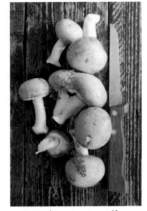

Onions: Onions are high in chromium, copper, folate, manganese, phosphorus, potassium and vitamins B6 and C. These nutrients help to enhance immune system function. The vegetable also supports healthy bones and connective tissue by keeping joints lubricated.

Salmon: Salmon is a great anti-inflammatory food due to the high amounts of protein and omega-3 fatty acids it contains. The omega-3s help reduce triglycerides and cholesterol and lower blood pressure. Salmon reduces inflammation in bones, joints and muscles. Just 4 ounces of salmon contains 87% of the recommended daily amount of omega-3. Eating 2-3 servings of salmon each week provides you with the same benefits as a fish oil capsule.

Four Week Menu with Recipes

SIMPLE BANANA PANCAKES - BREAKFAST DAY 1

Yield: 1 serving

Ingredients

1 Tbsp coconut oil
1 banana
2 eggs

Directions:

Smash the banana and puree in a blender or food processor. Add two eggs to the mixture and combine. Put small amount of oil in a skillet until warm, then spoon in batter. When it starts to bubble, flip the pancake. Keep going until you have a stack.

SPAGHETTI SQUASH AND SAUCE - LUNCH DAY 1

Yield: 8 servings

Ingredients

1/4 cup water
1 spaghetti squash, halved
  lengthwise and seeded
1 1/2 lbs ground beef
1 white onion, diced
1/2 cup + 1 Tbsp olive oil
1 cup mushrooms, sliced
1 zucchini, diced
1 red bell pepper, diced
1 green bell pepper, diced
3 – 8 oz cans crushed
  tomatoes
1/4 cup basil
1/4 cup oregano
1/4 cup thyme
1 Tbsp red pepper flakes

Directions:

Preheat oven to 400°F. Place squash face-down on a baking dish and roast for 30 – 40 minutes, or until tender. Brown beef with the onions in a skillet over medium high heat. Drain grease and remove from heat. Heat 1 Tbsp of olive oil and sauté mushrooms, zucchini, bell peppers, crushed tomatoes, basil, oregano and thyme for about 10 minutes. Add the ground beef and onion to the skillet and simmer on low heat until the squash is finished cooking, stirring occasionally. Shred the inside of the hot spaghetti squash into strands with a fork. Top each portion with a Tbsp of olive oil and a generous amount of meat sauce.

Yield: 6 servings

Ingredients

7 cups tomato, diced
2 small onions, diced
1/2 yellow summer squash, diced
4 medium zucchini, thinly sliced lengthwise
1 egg
1/2 cup coconut milk
1 lb ground turkey
1/4 cup + 1 1/2 tsp olive oil
1/2 tsp honey
18 large basil leaves, chopped
1 3/4 tsp salt
1/4 tsp pepper
1 tsp garlic, minced

Directions:

In a large saucepan, heat 1/2 tsp olive oil on medium to high heat. Sauté the onion and 1 tsp salt for 2 minutes, then add the garlic for 1 minute. Reduce to medium heat and add tomatoes and honey. Cook for 20 minutes, or until the sauce thickens slightly.

In a separate pan warm 1 Tbsp olive oil and brown the turkey. After several minutes, add the onion, 1/2 tsp salt and 1/4 tsp pepper. After meat is finished cooking, remove from heat and drain grease. Add fresh basil.

In a small saucepan heat 1/2 tsp olive oil. Sauté the chopped onion, squash, 1/4 tsp salt and 1/2 tsp minced garlic for 3 – 4 minutes. Add 1/4 cup coconut milk and allow to boil. Reduce heat and allow to simmer for 2 minutes. Put this mixture into a blender with an additional 1/4 cup coconut milk. Puree until smooth and add 1 egg. Mix until blended.

Grease the inside of a slow cooker and add 3/4 cup of tomato mixture. Make sure it covers the bottom of the pot. On top of the sauce, place 5 zucchini slices side by side. Layer on about 1/2 cup of the coconut milk mixture and 3/4 cup of the tomato mixture. Repeat the process and end with the marinara sauce on top. Cover and cook on high for 90 minutes. Take off the lid and remove excess liquid from the slow cooker with a baster or ladle. Put the liquid in a frying pan and bring it to a boil. Reduce heat and let it simmer about 5 minutes, or until it becomes creamy. Pour this sauce over the lasagna in the slow cooker and serve.

EGG CUPS - BREAKFAST DAY 2

Yield: 3 servings

Ingredients

6 eggs
12 slices prosciutto
Salt and pepper to taste
Parsley for garnish

Directions:

Preheat oven to 400°F. Take a muffin tin and lightly grease 6 of the cups. Put two pieces of the prosciutto into each of the cups; it is important that there are no holes or the egg will leak through. Place one egg into each cup and season with salt and pepper to taste. Bake for 15 minutes. Let sit for 3 – 5 minutes before serving. Garnish with parsley, if desired.

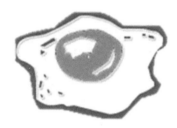

CHICKEN KABOBS: LUNCH DAY 2

Yield: 4 servings

Ingredients

1 lb boneless, skinless chicken
    breast, diced
2 garlic cloves, crushed
2 Tbsp ground cumin
2 Tbsp sesame oil
1/2 tsp salt
Metal skewers

Directions:

In a bowl, mix together the garlic, cumin, sesame oil and sea salt. Mix in the chicken, making sure each piece is coated with the mixture. Cover and place in a refrigerator or sealed container for two hours (or overnight). Line the chicken on a skewer, adding cut veggies if desired, and grill until chicken is fully cooked.

PESTO BAKED SALMON - DINNER DAY 2

Yield: 2 servings

Ingredients

2 medium-sized salmon filets
1/4 cup chopped walnuts
5 garlic cloves
1 jalapeno pepper
2 Tbsp olive oil
1 Tbsp chopped basil
3 Tbsp + 1/2 tsp chopped
  spinach
Salt and pepper to taste

Directions:

Preheat oven to 450°F. Sprinkle olive oil, salt and pepper on salmon. Place on a lined baking sheet and bake for 12 – 15 minutes. Add garlic, jalapeno, spinach, basil and walnut pieces in a food processor until combined. Add olive oil, salt and pepper and puree until smooth.

When salmon is finished cooking top with mixture.

SQUASH AND EGG RINGS - BREAKFAST DAY 3

Yield: 3 – 4 servings (depending on squash size)

Ingredients

1 acorn squash
Olive oil
1 large egg for each slice of
  squash
Salt and pepper to taste
Fresh herbs

Directions:

Preheat the oven to 425°F. Slice the squash crosswise and remove all seeds and pulp. The rings should be about ¾" thick. Put foil on a baking sheet and spray with cooking oil. Line the rings on the sheet and lightly brush olive oil on the squash tops and insides. The rings will bake for about 20 minutes then need to be turned over and put back into the oven. Take the sheet out of the oven and crack an egg into the middle of each ring. Top with salt and pepper to taste and put the baking sheet back into the oven for 8–12 minutes. Take out when the whites are just about set (they will continue to cook a little more after you remove them from the oven). Lift from the baking sheet with a spatula and top with herbs if you like. Serve while still warm!

CABBAGE TACO WRAPS - LUNCH DAY 3

Yield: 2 – 4 servings

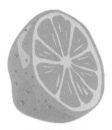 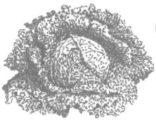 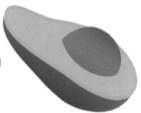

Ingredients

1 lb ground beef
Napa cabbage leaves
1/2 yellow onion, diced
1 – 14 oz can diced tomatoes
1 – 4 oz can diced green chilies
Juice of 1 1/2 limes
1 avocado
3 garlic cloves, minced
1/4 tsp garlic powder
1/4 tsp onion powder
1 tsp oregano
1 tsp cumin
1 tsp cayenne pepper
Salt and pepper to taste

Directions:

Cook beef in skillet over medium high heat. After halfway browned, add onion and minced garlic cloves. Once completely cooked, drain grease. Add 1/2 cup water to meat mixture and add oregano, cumin, salt, pepper, cayenne pepper, juice of 1 lime, tomatoes and green chilies. Reduce heat and allow mixture to simmer. Make guacamole by mashing the avocado and stirring in the garlic powder, onion powder, a pinch of cayenne pepper, juice from 1/2 lime and salt to taste. Clean the cabbage leaves and spoon the taco meat inside. Top with guacamole.

APPLE BACON PORK BURGERS - DINNER DAY 3

Yield: 3 servings

Ingredients
1 lb ground pork 6 – 8 bacon strips, cut into   1" pieces 1 apple, cored and diced 1 – 2 Tbsp rosemary Salt and pepper to taste

Directions:

Add the chopped bacon to a medium skillet and cook on medium heat. Once the bacon fat starts seeping out, add the diced apple and let cook for 5 – 7 minutes. Put the bacon and apples on a paper towel and allow to cool. Put the ground pork in a bowl and combine with rosemary, salt and pepper. Make a small ball of the pork and smash it with your thumbs into a very thin patty. Make another one just like it. Place a spoonful of bacon and apples on top of a patty and cover with another patty. Pinch the sides with your fingers to seal. You should be able to make about 3 burgers with 1 pound of pork. Next, reheat the skillet and add the burgers. Cook at least 5 minutes on each side, making sure that they are thoroughly cooked.

EGG CUPS - BREAKFAST DAY 4
SEE BREAKFAST DAY 2

Page 16

SPAGHETTI SQUASH AND SAUCE - LUNCH DAY 4
SEE LUNCH DAY 1

Page 14

Yield: 3 servings

Ingredients

1 1/2 lbs boneless, skinless chicken breast, diced into bite-sized pieces
2 carrots, diced
1/2 large head green cabbage, shredded
3 cups mushrooms
1 can coconut milk
1/2 cup chicken stock
1 Tbsp Thai curry paste
1 – 2 splashes fish sauce
1 – 2 splashes coconut aminos

Directions:

Mix coconut milk and curry in a large pot, stirring until well blended. Heat the mixture to a boil, and then reduce to a simmer for 5 minutes. Chop vegetables. Add carrots, chicken, fish sauce, chicken stock and aminos into the simmering curry. Mix together and continue simmering for 10 minutes. Put the cabbage and mushrooms into the mixture and cook 3 – 5 minutes.

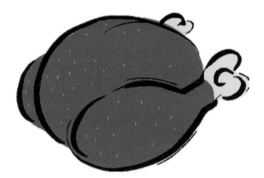

SIMPLE BANANA PANCAKES - BREAKFAST DAY 5
SEE BREAKFAST DAY 1

Page 14

SAUCY JOE'S - LUNCH DAY 5

Yield: 4 servings

Ingredients

2 Tbsp olive oil
1 onion, chopped
1 green bell pepper, chopped
2 garlic cloves, minced
1 lb ground beef
1 – 15 oz can tomato sauce
1 Tbsp chili powder
1/2 tsp ground cumin

Directions:

Heat oil in a large skillet on medium high and sauté onion, pepper and garlic about 10 minutes, or until tender. Add the ground beef and cook 8 – 10 more minutes while the meat begins to brown. Pour in tomato sauce, chili powder and cumin and continue cooking until beef is cooked through. Drain grease and remove from heat. Eat alone or serve inside bell peppers or on top of vegetable spaghetti noodles.

CROCKPOT SQUASH AND BEEF STEW - DINNER DAY 5

Yield: 5 – 7 servings

Ingredients

2 – 3 lbs beef stew meat
1 medium butternut squash, cubed
1 medium leek, diced
1 large onion, diced
5 garlic cloves, minced
2 Tbsp Italian seasoning
1 qt beef stock
4 – 8 oz red cooking wine
3 – 4 oz sun dried tomatoes
Salt and pepper to taste

Directions:

In a large skillet sauté the onion, leek and garlic until about halfway done. Add the beef to the mixture and let it break down. Put all of this into a large slow cooker, along with the squash and seasonings. Pour red wine and beef broth into the slow cooker, covering all the ingredients. Cook on high for 5 – 7 hours or low for 7 – 9 hours.

SQUASH AND EGG RINGS - BREAKFAST DAY 6
SEE BREAKFAST DAY 3
Page 17

ASPARAGUS ROLL - LUNCH DAY 6
Yield: 2 servings

Ingredients
12 asparagus spears 1 1/2 tsp olive oil 4 thin slices smoked turkey

Directions:

Preheat oven to 400°F. Prepare the asparagus by cutting off the thick base of each spear. Put the spears on a plate and drizzle oil over them. Cut each turkey slice into 3 strips and wrap a strip around each asparagus spear, leaving the tip visible. Place the asparagus on a lined baking dish and put in the oven for 12 minutes, flipping halfway through.

TROPICAL CHICKEN - DINNER DAY 6
Yield: 4 servings

Ingredients
2 lbs chicken meat, cuts of choice 1/2 fresh pineapple, skinned, cored and cut into 1" pieces 1/2 fresh mango, skinned and cut into 1" pieces Juice from 1 lemon 2 Tbsp olive oil 1/2 tsp cayenne pepper

Directions:

Heat oven to 375°F. Rinse the chicken and put into a shallow baking dish. Puree the fruit, lemon juice, olive oil and cayenne in a blender. Pour the mixture over the chicken and cover the dish with foil. Cook for 45 minutes to one hour, depending on the thickness of your chicken. Serve with a vegetable or challenge approved side dish of your choice.

22

SWEET POTATO AND BACON HASH - BREAKFAST DAY 7

Yield: 2 servings

Ingredients

3 slices bacon, diced
1 small onion, finely chopped
1 large apple, cut into 1" cubes
1 tsp cinnamon
1 - 2 Tbsp coconut oil
1 large sweet potato, peeled and cut into 1" cubes
1 Tbsp fresh sage, minced

Directions:

Cook bacon in a skillet on medium-low heat. When crispy, take out of the pan and leave the grease. Put the onion, apples and cinnamon into the same skillet and keep cooking; after 7 minutes the mixture should be soft. Take mixture from the pan and place with the bacon, making sure to leave some fat in the pan. Cook the sweet potatoes in leftover fat for about 2 minutes, adding coconut oil if bacon fat is gone. Stir once, then keep cooking for another 8 minutes or until soft. Add bacon and apple mixture back to the pan and add the sage. Cook until warm, remove from heat and enjoy!

SPICY CHICKEN WRAPS - LUNCH DAY 7

Yield: 2 – 4 servings

Ingredients

1 lb boneless, skinless chicken thighs
2 tsp chipotle powder
1/2 tsp garlic powder
1/2 tsp onion powder
2 Tbsp coconut oil
1 head romaine lettuce or napa cabbage
1 avocado, sliced
1/2 cup grape tomatoes, halved
2 Tbsp chopped green onion
Salt and pepper to taste

Directions:

Combine the chipotle powder, garlic powder, onion powder, salt and pepper in a bowl. Cut the chicken into thin strips and mix into the bowl. Melt the oil in a skillet over medium heat and add the chicken. Cook for 5 – 10 minutes, or until the chicken is cooked all the way through, turning when necessary. Serve with a lettuce or cabbage wrap and garnish with avocado, tomato and green onion.

TOM YUM SOUP - DINNER DAY 7

Yield: 4 servings

Ingredients

1 Tbsp ginger paste
1 Tbsp lemongrass paste
1 Tbsp cilantro
1 shallot, chopped
2 large chilies, seeded and
  chopped
1 Tbsp olive oil
2 Tbsp Thai fish sauce
2 quarts chicken stock
1 cup sliced mushrooms
9 cooked, shelled shrimp

Directions:

Combine ginger paste, lemongrass paste, cilantro, shallot, chilies, olive oil and fish sauce in a food processor until well combined. Put in a soup pot and add chicken stock. Bring to a boil and add mushrooms. Reduce heat to a simmer for 15 minutes. Add shrimp and cook for an additional 2 minutes.

EGG AND HAM WRAP - BREAKFAST DAY 8

Yield: 1 – 2 servings

Ingredients

1 Tbsp olive oil
5 eggs
4 - 8 thin slices of ham
1 tomato, diced
1/2 small onion, diced
1 red bell pepper, diced
1/4 teaspoon chili flakes
Sea salt and pepper to taste

Directions:

Warm oil in a pan over medium high heat, and cook onions, peppers and chili flakes for 6 minutes, or until soft. Add tomatoes to the pan and cook for two minutes. Whisk the eggs together and add to the skillet until completely cooked. Put the mixture in the center of the ham slices, rolling into a burrito-like shape. Place the rolls into pan and heat each roll until slightly brown.

Yield: 4 patties

Ingredients

2 Tbsp coconut oil
1 1/4 lbs ground turkey
2 large garlic cloves, minced
1" ginger root, grated
3 green onions, diced
1 bag broccoli slaw
1/2 cup almond butter
3 Tbsp coconut aminos or
   tamari soy sauce
1/2 cup chicken broth
1 tsp red pepper flakes
Salt and pepper to taste

Directions:

Mix together ground turkey, garlic, ginger, onions, salt and pepper in a bowl. Make 4 patties and set aside. Warm coconut oil in a pan over medium heat, add the patties and cook for 6 minutes. Flip patties and cook until brown, about 3 minutes. Put the lid on the pan and cook until patties are cooked to an internal temperature of 165°F. Place the almond butter and aminos in a small saucepan and warm over medium low heat. Stir continuously and gradually pour in broth until mixture is creamy. Put finished burgers on a plate, top with sauce and garnish with broccoli slaw.

Yield: 5 servings

Ingredients

2 1/2 lbs smoked bacon
3 handfuls fresh spinach,
   stems removed
1 lb mushrooms, sliced
1 large onion, chopped
2 garlic cloves, minced
2 Tbsp butter

Directions:

Cook the bacon until soft, not crispy, in a large skillet over medium heat. Add onion and cook for 5 minutes. When the onion is soft, add garlic and mushrooms and cook for 8 minutes. Stir the spinach and butter into the mixture and cover for 4 minutes, or until the spinach is finished.

❯ EGGS AND VEGGIES - BREAKFAST DAY 9 ❮

Yield: 1 serving

Ingredients

1/2 Tbsp coconut oil
1 1/2 cups veggies of choice 3 eggs
1/4 avocado, diced for garnish
Salt and pepper to taste

Directions:

Warm oil in a skillet over medium heat and sauté veggies for 3 minutes, or until tender. Whisk eggs in a bowl and add to skillet. Mix together and season with salt and pepper. When eggs are cooked, plate and garnish with the avocado.

❯ SALMON PATTIES - LUNCH DAY 9 ❮

Yield: 6 servings

Ingredients

1 large sweet potato, cooked and mashed
2/3 cup almond meal
1/3 cup parsley, chopped
2 Tbsp onion, chopped
1 Tbsp lemon juice
1/2 - 1 Tbsp hot sauce
1/2 Tbsp salt
1 tsp cumin
1 1/4 tsp paprika
1/2 tsp pepper
2 eggs
2 – 15 oz cans of salmon
2 Tbsp coconut oil

Directions:

In a large bowl, mix the sweet potato, almond meal, parsley, onion, lemon juice, hot sauce, salt, cumin, paprika, pepper and eggs. Drain the liquid from the cans of salmon, and mix the salmon with the other ingredients. With a 1/3 measuring cup, make salmon patties and put them on a tray lined with parchment paper. Put the patties in the refrigerator for at least 30 minutes (or freeze if they will not be cooked within 12 - 24 hours). Heat 1 Tbsp oil in a large frying pan over medium high heat. Once the pan is hot, carefully place the salmon patties in the skillet and cook for 4 minutes on each side. You will need approximately 1 Tbsp of oil for every 6 patties. Serve while hot.

Yield: 2 – 4 servings

Ingredients

1 cup almond flour
3 Tbsp almond butter
2 eggs, beaten
1/2 tsp sea salt
3 tsp olive oil
1/2 cup onion, diced
4 mushrooms, sliced
1 large Italian sausage, cut into
    1/2" slices
2 garlic cloves, minced
1 bell pepper, diced
1/2 cup tomato sauce
1/2 tsp dried oregano
1/2 tsp fennel seed
1/2 cup cherry tomatoes,
    halved

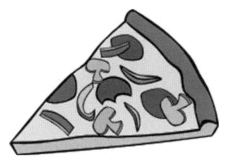

Directions:

Preheat oven to 350°F. In a small bowl, combine the almond flour, almond butter, eggs and sea salt. Spread 2 tsp of oil on a baking sheet and spread the mixture on top, making a 1/4" thick crust. Put the sheet in the oven for 10 minutes. Warm a large skillet over medium high heat and add the remaining olive oil, onions, mushrooms and slices sausage. Cook until the sausage is browned and the onions are translucent. Remove this mixture from the skillet into a separate bowl. Put the garlic and bell pepper into the skillet and sauté – do not cook them all the way, as they will be cooking more in the oven. Take the crust from the oven and spread the tomato sauce on top. Top with the sausage mixture, sautéed veggies, oregano and fennel seed. Bake the pizza for 20 – 30 minutes. Be careful when taking the slices off the sheet as the dough may be soft. Garnish with sliced tomatoes and serve.

Yield: 2 servings

Ingredients

1 Tbsp olive oil
3/4 lb sausage
1 acorn squash, halved and
   seeded
2 eggs
½ yellow onion, diced
1 garlic clove, minced
Salt and pepper to taste

Directions:

Preheat oven to 375°F. Lay squash face down on baking sheet and bake for 20 - 25 minutes. Warm oil in large skillet over medium heat and cook garlic and onion for 5 minutes. Add sausage until completely cooked. With a spoon, scoop out squash, leaving 1/4" near the skin. Combine the scooped squash with the mixture and add to squash skin. Using a spoon, make a place for your egg. Add the egg and put the squash bowls back on baking sheet and into the oven for 10 – 15 minutes, or until egg is finished.

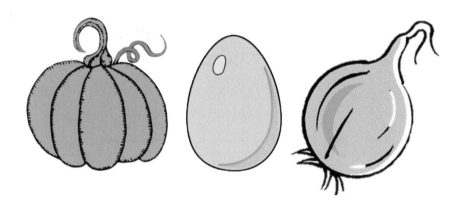

SPICY CHICKEN SOUP - LUNCH DAY 10

Yield: 6 servings

Ingredients

2 Tbsp coconut oil
1 onion, finely chopped
6 garlic cloves, minced
6 boneless, skinless chicken
   thighs, cut into 1/2" pieces
2 canned chipotle chilies in
   adobo sauce, finely chopped
2 Tbsp adobo sauce
6 cups chicken broth
1 cup carrots, chopped
1/2 cup cilantro, chopped
Juice of 2 limes
1 avocado, thinly sliced
Salt and pepper to taste

Directions:

Heat the oil over medium high heat in a large pot. Lower the heat and add the onion and garlic. After 7 minutes, stir the onion to the side of the pot. Turn the heat on high and add the chicken for about 5 minutes, or until the chicken is golden. Add carrots, chipotle chilies and adobo sauce and stir. Pour in the chicken broth and simmer for 15 minutes on low heat. Right before removing from heat stir in the cilantro and lime juice. Serve in bowls and garnish with avocado.

EASY FISH FILETS - DINNER DAY 10

Yield: 4 servings

Ingredients

2 Tbsp olive oil
1 onion, thinly sliced
2 garlic cloves, minced
1 – 14.5 oz can diced
   tomatoes
1/2 cup black olives, pitted and
   sliced
1 Tbsp chopped parsley
1/2 cup dry white wine
1 lb cod filets

Directions:

Heat oil over medium heat in a large skillet. Sauté the onions and garlic, then add the tomatoes, olives, parsley and wine. After simmering for 5 minutes, put the filets in the sauce. Continue to simmer for 5 minutes, or until the fish turns white.

EGG AND HAM WRAP - DAY 11 BREAKFAST
SEE BREAKFAST DAY 8
Page 24

CHICKEN CHIMICHURRI - DAY 11 LUNCH

Yield: 6 – 8 servings

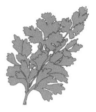

Ingredients

Chicken
8 bone-in chicken thighs
1 1/4 cup chimichurri sauce, divided
Lettuce

Chimichurri Sauce
1 cup fresh parsley
3/4 cup olive oil
3 Tbsp lemon juice
2 Tbsp red wine vinegar
3 garlic cloves, peeled
1 tsp dried oregano
1 tsp salt
1/2 tsp chipotle chili flakes
1/4 tsp pepper

Directions:

Make the sauce by pulsing all ingredients in the food processor until the parsley and garlic are finely chopped.

Place the chicken in a shallow pan and marinate with 1/3 cup of the sauce for a minimum of 30 minutes. Preheat the grill and cook for 10 – 13 minutes, flipping halfway through. Cover your plate with lettuce, add chicken and top with the remaining sauce.

PAD THAI - DAY II DINNER

Yield: 2 servings

Ingredients

2 skinless chicken breasts, cubed
4 yellow squash, julienned or spiralized
1/4 cup almond butter
1 Tbsp sesame oil
3 garlic cloves, minced
1 sprig shallot, minced
1/2 cup coconut aminos
1/4 tsp fish sauce
Juice of 1/2 lime
1 tsp salt
1/3 cup raw macadamia nuts, chopped
1/8 cup cilantro for garnish
1 tsp red pepper flakes

Directions:

Peel squash and put the julienned "noodles" into a steamer basket for 5 – 8 minutes. In a bowl, mix the almond butter with coconut aminos, fish sauce, juice from 1/2 lime and salt. Heat a wok to high heat and add the sesame oil. Place the cubed chicken in the wok and stir fry until it is white. Stir in the shallot, garlic and red pepper flakes. Stir fry for 1 minute, then mix in the nuts and continue cooking for 2 minutes. Add the fish sauce and stir until everything is coated. Lower heat and combine with squash. Garnish with cilantro.

SAUSAGE STUFFED SQUASH - BREAKFAST DAY I2
SEE BREAKFAST DAY I0

Page 28

EGG SALAD AND AVOCADO WRAP - LUNCH DAY 12

Yield: 2 servings

Ingredients

4 hard-boiled eggs, mashed
1 very ripe avocado
1 Tbsp parsley
4 romaine lettuce leaves
Salt and pepper to taste

Directions:

Mix together the hard boiled eggs, avocado, parsley, salt and pepper. Spread into each of the lettuce leaves and roll.

BEEF STIR FRY WITH CASHEWS - DINNER DAY 12

Yield: 3 – 4 servings

Directions:

Ingredients

1 cup coconut aminos
1/2 cup orange juice
3 Tbsp honey
1 tsp fish sauce
2 garlic cloves, minced
1 tsp fresh ginger, grated
1/2 tsp red pepper flakes
3 Tbsp arrowroot powder
1 lb flank steak, thinly sliced
  against the grain
3 crowns of broccoli, cut into
  florets
2 Tbsp coconut oil
1/2 cup toasted cashews
Salt and pepper to taste

Make a marinade by whisking together coconut aminos, orange juice, honey, fish sauce, garlic, ginger, red pepper flakes, arrowroot powder, salt and pepper. Pour mixture over the steak slices and cover in the refrigerator for at least 30 minutes. Heat 1 Tbsp of oil in a large pan over medium heat. When warmed, add the broccoli and sprinkle with salt. Cook to your preference, then remove from the pan. Put the pan back on the stove on high heat and add another

Tbsp of oil. Place the marinated steak into the pan and cook until the pink is almost gone. Put the broccoli back in the pan and add the cashews. Stir together all ingredients and continue cooking for 1 minute.

SEE BREAKFAST DAY 9
Page 26

SMOKY SHRIMP SLAW - LUNCH DAY 13
Yield: 4 servings

Ingredients

1/2 head green cabbage, shredded
1/4 cup carrots, shredded
2/3 cup celery, chopped
2/3 cup red radishes, thinly sliced
1/4 cup green onion, chopped
1/2 cup flat-leaf parsley, chopped
1 1/2 – 2 pounds raw shrimp, peeled and deveined
4 strips bacon, cooked and chopped
3 Tbsp olive oil
1 tsp smoked paprika
1 Tbsp minced garlic
Salt and pepper to taste

Directions:

Prepare slaw by combining the cabbage, carrots, celery, radishes, green onion and parsley in a large bowl and set aside. In another bowl, combine the shrimp, oil, paprika, salt, pepper and garlic. Sauté the shrimp over medium heat in a large, nonstick frying pan. Cook until they are opaque and remove from heat. Mix the shrimp with the slaw and top with chopped bacon.

GRILLED ORIENTAL RIBS - DINNER DAY 13

Yield: 6 servings

Ingredients

6 lbs pork baby back ribs (cut into 6 portions)
1 Tbsp Chinese spice blend
1 tsp curry powder
1/2 tsp paprika
1/2 tsp ground coriander
3 Tbsp sesame oil
1/3 cup coconut aminos
1/2 tsp fish sauce
2 garlic cloves, minced
1 Tbsp ginger root, minced

Directions:

Place the ribs into two large soup pots that are 2/3 full of water. Once they come to a boil, cover and par boil for 30 minutes. Drain the ribs from the pots and cool on a baking sheet. After they are cooled, sprinkle with the Chinese spice blend, curry powder, paprika and ground coriander and cover with foil. Place in the refrigerator for 1 hour.

Whisk together sesame oil, aminos, fish sauce, garlic and ginger and set the bowl aside. Soak hickory chips in water for 1 hour. When finished, put the chips in a smoker box. Place the box on a grill set on low heat. Grill the ribs for 20 minutes and baste with the glaze. Keep cooking over low heat for 15 minutes.

OAT-FREE OATMEAL - BREAKFAST DAY 14

Yield: 1 serving

Ingredients

2 Tbsp unsweetened coconut flakes
1 Tbsp pumpkin seeds
1 Tbsp flax seed
2 tsp chia seed
1 Tbsp walnuts
1/2 tsp cinnamon
1/2 - 3/4 cup hot water
7 – 10 drops liquid stevia or honey
2 - 4 Tbsp coconut or almond milk
1/2 cup berries of choice

Directions:

Grind coconut, pumpkin seeds, flax seed, chia seed, walnuts and cinnamon in a coffee grinder or food processor and put the mixture into a bowl. Cover with hot water and allow it to thicken by letting it sit for a few minutes. Add milk, stevia drops and berries and mix until well combined.

STEAK FAJITAS - LUNCH DAY 14

Yield: 3 – 4 servings

Ingredients

3 garlic cloves, minced
1 1/2 lbs flank steak
1 Tbsp butter
1 onion, diced
1 bell pepper, diced
Salt and pepper to taste

Directions:

Preheat the grill to medium high heat. Rub the garlic on the steak and sprinkle with salt. Grill for about 10 minutes, flipping halfway. Set aside when finished. Warm the butter in a pan over medium high heat and sauté the onion and peppers until they are hot. Plate the vegetables. Cut the steak against the grain and lay on top of the veggies.

SPICY GRILLED SALMON - DINNER DAY 14

Yield: 2 servings

Ingredients

2 salmon filets
2 pinches salt
1 Tbsp fresh thyme
1/4 tsp ginger
2 pinches cayenne pepper
2 pinches cumin
Olive oil, enough to make a
    paste
Ground black pepper to taste

Directions:

Heat the grill to medium. Make spice mixture by crushing the garlic and mixing in the seasonings. To make a paste of the spice mix add in approximately 2 Tbsp oil. Get a large sheet of foil and roll up each of the sides to make a tray. Lay the salmon skin-down on the tray and massage the paste into the top of the salmon. Place the foil on the grill, loosely cover with more foil and close the grill. Cook until the salmon is warm throughout and a little pink in the center, with an internal temperature of at least 135°F. It is difficult to give an exact time on this because it will depend on your grill and the size of the filets. Serve with sautéed veggies of your choice.

MEXICAN FRITTATA - BREAKFAST DAY 15

Yield: 4 – 6 servings

Ingredients

1 lb ground beef
2 sweet potatoes, shredded
1 small yellow onion, diced
6 eggs, whisked
2 garlic cloves, minced
1 Tbsp olive oil
1 – 14 oz can gluten free
   enchilada sauce
1 tsp chili powder
1/2 tsp cumin
1/2 tsp oregano
Salt and pepper to taste

Directions:

Preheat oven to 450°F. Warm olive oil in skillet over medium heat and sauté garlic and onion until onion is soft. Brown beef in pan, mixing it with onion and garlic while cooking. Mix in seasonings when the beef is almost finished. Put shredded sweet potatoes on top of the meat mixture. Flatten the sweet potatoes, pour the enchilada sauce over the top and cover for 8 – 10 minutes, or until sweet potatoes soften. Remove from heat. Mix in eggs and put the skillet into the oven for 25 – 30 minutes. (If your skillet is not oven-proof, move mixture to a different baking pan).

SPICY CHICKEN SOUP - LUNCH DAY 15
SEE LUNCH DAY 10

APPLE PORK CHOPS - DINNER DAY 15

Yield: 4 servings

Ingredients

4 bone-in pork chops
3 Tbsp coconut oil
2 large onion, sliced
4 apples, cored and sliced
Salt and pepper to taste

Directions:

Heat 2 Tbsp coconut oil in a large pan over medium high heat and cook the pork chops for 5 minutes on each side. Remove fromthe pan and lower heat to medium low. Cook the apple and onion slices with 1 Tbsp of coconut oil for 4 minutes. Cover the pork chops with the warm apple and onion mixture.

Yield: 4 – 6 servings

Ingredients

1 small zucchini, shredded
1 small squash, shredded
1 small carrot, shredded
1/2 yellow onion, shredded
1 cup almond flour
2 eggs, whisked
2 garlic cloves, minced
1 tsp dried basil
1 tsp dried parsley
2 Tbsp coconut oil
Salt and pepper to taste
Avocado, diced, for garnish
Green onion, diced, for garnish

Directions:

Shred vegetables with a food processor or cheese shredder. Combine the shredded vegetables with almond flour, eggs, garlic, basil, parsley, salt and pepper. Flatten out 6 – 7" "pancakes" from the mixture. Warm coconut oil in a large pan over medium high heat. Place as many pancakes as fit comfortably in the pan and cook 5 – 7 minutes on each side, or until brown. Plate and garnish with diced avocado and green onions.

Yield: 2 – 4 servings

Ingredients

2 cups cooked, chopped
  chicken breast
2 stalks celery, chopped
1 small apple, chopped
2 green onions, chopped
1/4 cup walnuts, chopped
2 Tbsp Paleo mayonnaise
1/8 tsp paprika
Salt and pepper to taste

Directions:

Mix the chopped chicken, celery, apple, green onions and walnuts. Add mayonnaise to hold the ingredients together. Add salt, pepper and paprika to your liking.

CROCKPOT ASIAN PORK - DINNER DAY 16

Yield: 4 servings

Ingredients

3 lbs pork shoulder, cubed
1/4 cup sesame oil
6 garlic cloves, minced
1/4 cup rice vinegar
2 Tbsp fresh ginger, grated
1/4 cup chives, chopped
1/2 cup coconut aminos

Directions:

Combine the oil, vinegar, ginger, chives and aminos in a large bowl. Mix the cubed pork until coated with the dressing. Place mixture into a slow cooker and cook on low. After 6 hours, remove the pork and put in a large baking dish. Broil for 8 – 10 minutes so that the pork is brown and crispy.

SAUSAGE AND BLUEBERRY SWEET POTATOES BREAKFAST DAY 17

Yield: 4 servings

Ingredients

2 sweet potatoes, halved
1 cup blueberries
1 lb sausage
1 egg, whisked
Salt and pepper to taste

Directions:

Preheat the oven to 400°F. Place sweet potatoes face down on a lined baking sheet and cook for 25 – 30 minutes. Brown the sausage in a pan over medium heat, then add the blueberries, salt and pepper. Drain excess fat from the pan. Place mixture into a bowl and mix in the whisked egg. Allow the sweet potatoes to cool after removing them from the oven and remove the middles with a spoon. There should be about 1/4" of the potato remaining in the skin. Place the sweet potatoes back on the baking sheet and spoon in the sausage mixture. Bake for 6 – 8 minutes and allow to cool before eating.

TURKEY WRAPPED VEGGIES - LUNCH DAY 17

Yield: 1 serving

Ingredients

4 turkey slices
1 avocado, sliced
Vinaigrette dressing to taste
1/2 cup shredded carrots

Directions:

Take two turkey slices and overlap them. Put half of the shredded carrots and avocado slices on top and spoon a bit of vinaigrette dressing over the top. Use the turkey slices as your wrap and roll them up. Repeat with the remaining ingredients.

PALEO MEATLOAF - DINNER DAY 17

Yield: 3 – 4 servings

Ingredients

1 lb ground beef
1 yellow onion, diced
1 roasted red pepper, diced
1 cup tomato sauce
1 egg, whisked
2 Tbsp olive oil
3/4 cup almond flour
2 tsp dried basil
2 tsp dried thyme
2 tsp dried parsley
Salt and pepper to taste

Directions:

Preheat oven to 400°F. Pour olive oil in a medium pan over medium heat and add onion and peppers. Remove from heat when onions become translucent. In a bowl, mix the ground beef, onion and pepper mixture, 1/4 cup tomato sauce, egg, almond flour, 1 tsp dried basil, 1 tsp dried thyme and 1 tsp dried parsley.

Use your hands to mix the ingredients and put into a bread pan and form into a loaf. Bake for 35 – 40 minutes. Combine 3/4 cup tomato sauce, 1 tsp dried basil, 1 tsp dried thyme and 1 tsp dried parsley in a pan and heat until it reaches a slight boil. After the meatloaf has cooled, top with the sauce.

ZUCCHINI SQUASH FLAPJACKS - BREAKFAST DAY 18
SEE BREAKFAST DAY 16

Page 37

SESAME GINGER STEAK SALAD - LUNCH DAY 18

Yield: 2 servings

Ingredients

10 oz sirloin steak
1 1/2 cups shredded cabbage
1/4 bell pepper, thinly sliced
1 radish, thinly sliced
1 medium carrot, shredded
8 grape tomatoes, halved
1/2 navel orange, chopped
1/8 cup slivered almonds
1/2 green onion, chopped
4 Tbsp coconut aminos
2 Tbsp fish sauce
2 Tbsp sesame oil
2 tsp sesame seed
1 tsp salt and pepper
Red pepper flakes to taste
1 garlic clove, minced
1/2 Tbsp garlic powder
1 Tbsp ginger, minced

Directions:

Make a marinade for the steak by whisking together 2 Tbsp coconut aminos, fish sauce, minced garlic, 1/2 Tbsp ginger, 1 Tbsp salt and pepper and red pepper flakes to taste. Let the steak refrigerate in the marinade for 3 hours or overnight. Make the salad dressing by combining garlic powder, 1/2 Tbsp ginger, sesame oil, 2 Tbsp coconut aminos, sesame seeds, salt, pepper and red pepper flakes. Refrigerate dressing until ready for use. Preheat the grill to high heat and cook the steak for 8 – 10 minutes, flipping halfway through. Set the steak to the side. Mix cabbage, bell pepper, radish, carrot, tomatoes and orange in a bowl. Slice the steak into thin strips and add to the top of the salad with the almonds and green onion. Add dressing to taste.

SWEET POTATO AND LEMON CHICKEN DINNER DAY 18

Yield: 4 servings

Ingredients

1/4 cup olive oil
4 chicken breasts
1 1/2 sweet potatoes, cubed
Juice of 1 large lemon
1 large lemon, sliced
2 Tbsp rosemary
5 garlic cloves, minced

Directions:

Preheat the oven to 450°F. Warm the olive oil in a skillet over medium high heat. Season chicken with salt and pepper and put into the skillet. Add sweet potatoes and cook 8 – 10 minutes, or until chicken is browned. Put the mixture into a roasting pan and top with lemon juice, lemon slices, rosemary and garlic. Bake for 40 – 45 minutes.

MEXICAN FRITTATA - BREAKFAST DAY 19

SEE BREAKFAST DAY 15

Page 36

SALMON SEAWEED WRAP - LUNCH DAY 19

Yield: 1 serving

Ingredients

1 toasted seaweed sheet
1/4 avocado, sliced
2 oz smoked salmon
2 cucumber slices
1 thin lemon slice

Directions:

Lay the seaweed on a plate or cutting board. Put the avocado, salmon, cucumber and lemon over it, and use the seaweed as a wrap for all the ingredients.

SPICY CROCKPOT PULLED PORK - DINNER DAY 19

Yield: 6 – 8 servings

Ingredients

2 lbs pork roast (excess fat trimmed)
3 garlic cloves, peeled
2 yellow onions, diced
2 red bell peppers, diced
2 – 14 oz cans fire roasted tomatoes
1 – 14 oz can tomato sauce
1/2 cup hot sauce
3 Tbsp smoked paprika
2 Tbsp garlic powder
2 Tbsp cumin
2 tsp cayenne
1 Tbsp red pepper flakes
Avocado, sliced for garnish

Directions:

Place the roast in the slow cooker. With a knife, make 3 holes in the roast and put the peeled garlic in each hole. Pour the hot sauce over the meat and top with all spices. Cover the roast with onions, peppers, tomatoes and tomato sauce. Cover and cook for 8 – 10 hours on low heat. Shred the pork and garnish with avocado.

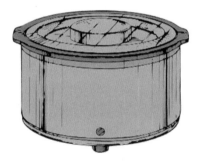

SAUSAGE AND BLUEBERRY SWEET POTATOES
BREAKFAST DAY 20
SEE BREAKFAST DAY 17

Page 38

42

Yield: 8 servings

Ingredients
4 cups broccoli, chopped and steamed
2 cups chicken or beef broth
4 cups cauliflower, chopped and steamed
4 – 6 garlic cloves, roasted
4 slices of bacon, cooked and chopped
Salt and pepper to taste

Directions:

Add 3 cups broccoli, 3 cups cauliflower, broth, garlic, salt and pepper to a blender. Blend on medium high until pureed. Place mixture in a large pot on the stove over medium heat and add the remaining broccoli and cauliflower. Stir the contents to blend and add salt and pepper to taste. Simmer for 10 minutes, adding more stock if you prefer your soup thinner. Serve in bowls and top with chopped bacon.

Yield: 4 servings

Ingredients
1 lb ground beef
1 head of cauliflower, riced
16 oz jar tomato sauce
1 – 2 Tbsp olives or capers for garnish

Directions:

Heat a large pan over medium-high heat and cook the beef until brown, draining any fat. Stir in the cauliflower and tomato sauce. Simmer until the cauliflower is tender, approximately 5 minutes. When finished, top with olives or capers.

43

BANANA NUT SALAD - BREAKFAST DAY 21
Yield: 1 serving

Ingredients

1 banana, peeled and sliced
1 handful roasted cashews
1 handful coconut chips

Directions:

In a bowl, layer the bananas, cashews and coconut chips. Serve immediately.

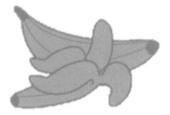

EGG SALAD WITH BLT - LUNCH DAY 21
Yield: 2 - 3 servings

Ingredients

6 hard-boiled eggs
1 avocado, peeled and pitted
2 tsp ground garlic
1 tsp salt
4 strips bacon, cooked and
    chopped
3/4 cup grape tomatoes,
    halved

Directions:

In a bowl, mash together your eggs, avocado, garlic and salt with a fork. Mix in the chopped bacon and tomatoes. Add additional seasoning to taste.

Yield: 4 servings

Ingredients

3/4 cup parsnips, peeled and grated
1 tsp onion salt
1 Tbsp olive oil
1 slice bacon
1/2 lb zucchini, sliced
1/4 lb mushrooms, sliced
1 celery stalk, diced
1 tsp coconut oil
1/2 red onion, diced
1 1/4 lb ground turkey
2 green onions, sliced
1 Tbsp Italian seasoning
1 tsp celery salt
1/2 tsp pepper
8 egg whites
1/2 cup parsley, chopped

Directions:

Preheat oven to 450°F. Mix the parsnips, onion salt and olive oil in a bowl. Warm a large pan over medium heat and cook bacon slice. Remove the bacon to cool. Sauté the zucchini, mushrooms and celery in the bacon fat until soft. In a separate pan, warm coconut oil over medium high heat and mix the ground turkey, onions, Italian seasoning, celery salt and pepper. Continue cooking until the turkey is completely done. Mix the meat and vegetables into one pan and stir until combined. Let the mixture cool for 5 minutes. In a separate bowl, whisk 4 egg whites and 1/4 cup parsley and add to the meat and veggie mixture. Whisk the remaining egg whites and parsley and set aside. Grease an 8x8" baking dish with olive oil and pour in the meat and veggie mix. Put the egg and parsley mix over the top and crumble the bacon over it all. Bake about 25 minutes, or until the top starts to brown.

EGGS WITH PESTO - BREAKFAST DAY 22

Yield: 2 servings

Ingredients
1 Tbsp coconut oil
4 eggs
1 – 2 Tbsp pesto

Directions

Warm coconut oil in a skillet over medium heat. Scramble eggs very slowly by cracking them directly into the pan and combining the yolks and the whites so that you can still see a color difference. After cooking for 1 minute, gently mix in the pesto. Keep scrambling the eggs until no longer runny.

HAM AND CUCUMBER ROLL UP - LUNCH DAY 22

Yield: 2 servings

Ingredients
6 slices thick-cut ham
1 cucumber, peeled
6 green onions
3 tsp paleo mayonnaise
1 jalapeno, diced
1 tsp dill
Toothpicks

Directions:

Slice the peeled cucumber lengthwise and cut each half lengthwise into four strips. These strips will be your "wraps". Mix the mayonnaise, jalapeno, and dill in a bowl. Put a slice of ham on a plate and spread the mayo mixture onto the ham slice. Roll the cucumber around the ham and onion. Hold together with a toothpick.

"SUNDAY" CHICKEN DINNER - DINNER DAY 22

Yield: 8 – 10 servings

Ingredients

4-5 lb whole chicken
Salt

Directions:

Preheat the oven to 450°F. Rinse the chicken well. Take paper towels and dry the chicken inside (the cavity) and out, then put it in a roasting pan. Season with the sea salt over the entire chicken, even inside the cavity. Cook for an hour or until thoroughly cooked to 165°F internal temperature. Serve with a vegetable or challenge-approved side of your choice.

SAUSAGE MUFFINS - BREAKFAST DAY 23

Yield: 4 servings

Ingredients

2-3 chicken sausage patties, cooked and chopped
1 red bell pepper, chopped
1/4 yellow onion, chopped
8 eggs, whisked
2 garlic cloves, minced
1/4 tsp garlic powder
1/8 tsp red pepper flakes
Salt and pepper to taste
Avocado, sliced for garnish
2 Tbsp olive oil or non-stick cooking spray

Directions:

Preheat oven to 325°F. Combine the sausage, pepper, onion, eggs, garlic cloves, garlic powder, red pepper flakes, salt and pepper. Pour mixture into 8 – 10 greased muffin tins. Bake for 35 – 40 minutes. Plate and garnish with avocado slices.

SIMPLE SALMON SALAD - LUNCH DAY 23

Yield: 2 servings

Ingredients

2 cans wild salmon, drained
2 cucumbers, diced
1 yellow onion, chopped
1 large tomato, chopped
1 avocado, chopped
5 – 6 Tbsp olive oil
Juice of 2 lemons
2 Tbsp fresh dill, chopped
Salt and pepper to taste
Lettuce leaves for serving

Directions:

Put the salmon in a bowl and mash with a fork. Mix in lemon juice, olive oil, cucumbers, onions, tomato and avocado. Season with fresh dill, salt and pepper to taste. Lay lettuce leaves on a plate and top with the mixture.

SWEET POTATO SOUP - DINNER DAY 23

Yield: 3 – 4 servings

Ingredients

2 sweet potatoes, diced
1/2 onion, sliced
1 – 14 oz can coconut milk
1 cup vegetable broth
2 garlic cloves
1 Tbsp dried basil
Salt and pepper to taste

Directions:

Place all ingredients into a slow cooker and mix together. Turn on high for 3 hours. Once cooked, pour the mixture in a blender or food processor and puree until smooth.

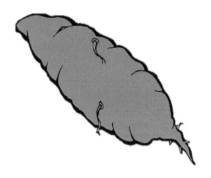

Yield: 3 servings

Ingredients

2 eggs
1/4 cup water
1 cup beets, chopped
1 cup turnips, chopped
1 cup Vidalia onion, chopped
2 Tbsp olive oil
1 Tbsp rosemary, minced
1 Tbsp garlic, minced
1 tsp coconut oil
Salt and pepper to taste

Directions:

Preheat oven to 400°F. Mix the beets, turnips, onions and olive oil in a bowl until well combined and spread onto a baking sheet. Sprinkle the mixture with salt, pepper and rosemary. Put baking sheet into the oven for 30 minutes, taking out after 20 minutes to mix in the garlic. Warm coconut oil over medium heat and crack an egg directly into the pan. After cooking for 30 seconds, pour in 1/4 cup water and cover with a lid until egg is fully cooked. Plate the hash and top with an egg.

Yield: 2 servings

Ingredients

2 cups grape tomatoes, halved
3 cucumbers
1 yellow or orange bell pepper
1/2 red onion, diced
2 large, ripe avocados
1 – 2 jalapeno peppers, diced
1 garlic clove, minced
1 handful fresh cilantro, chopped
Zest from 1 lime
1/3 cup lime juice
1/4 cup olive oil
1 tsp salt
1/4 tsp cayenne pepper

Directions:

Slice the cucumber, avocado and bell pepper into medium pieces and place in a bowl with the tomatoes, onion, cilantro and garlic. Zest the lime over the bowl. In smaller bowl mix together the fresh lime juice, olive oil, salt and cayenne pepper. Add to the salad bowl and toss to mix well.

SAUSAGE BASIL STUFFED BELL PEPPERS
DINNER DAY 24

Yield: 2 servings

Ingredients

2 bell peppers, halved and cleaned
1 Tbsp bacon grease or coconut oil
1/2 large onion, diced
4 garlic cloves, minced
1/2 cup diced tomatoes
1 lb ground beef, turkey or chicken
6 basil leaves, chopped
Salt and pepper to taste

Directions:

Preheat oven to 375°F. Warm the bacon grease in a skillet and sauté the onions, salt and pepper until the onions are translucent. Add the tomatoes and garlic to the pan and simmer for 2 minutes. Add the ground meat until completely cooked and add basil. Fill each pepper half with the meat mixture and bake for 15 – 20 minutes.

SAUSAGE MUFFINS - BREAKFAST DAY 25
SEE BREAKFAST DAY 23

Page 47

TUNA STUFFED CUCUMBER - LUNCH DAY 25

Yield: 1 serving

Ingredients

15 oz can light tuna, drained
2 Tbsp paleo mayonnaise
2 Tbsp chives
1 cucumber
8 cherry tomatoes
Salt and pepper to taste

Directions:

Slice the cucumber in half lengthwise and use a spoon or melon baller to scrape out the insides. Save the outside of the cucumber, and put the inside in a bowl. Add the chives, tuna, salt, pepper and mayonnaise to the bowl and thoroughly mash the mixture together. Spoon into the outside of the cucumber and top with cherry tomatoes.

Yield: 2 servings

Ingredients

1 medium butternut squash,
  peeled and diced
2 large pork chops
2 apples, sliced
1 sweet onion, thinly sliced
1 red onion, thinly sliced
1/2 cup chicken broth
5 Tbsp coconut oil
2 Tbsp honey
1 tsp mustard powder
3 tsp cinnamon
1/4 tsp nutmeg
Salt and pepper to taste

Directions:

Preheat oven to 350°F. Combine the squash, broth, 1 Tbsp coconut oil, 1 tsp cinnamon, nutmeg and salt in a slow cooker and cook on high for 1 hour (or low for 2 hours). Warm 2 skillets over medium heat, adding 2 Tbsp of coconut oil to each. Add the onions to one skillet and apple slices to the other. Stir ingredients in each skillet until the contents are translucent. Add 1 Tbsp of honey and 1 tsp of cinnamon to each skillet, stir and cook until caramelized. Add the onions to the apple skillet. Add salt, pepper, 2 tsp of cinnamon and mustard powder to each side of the pork chops and put the chops in the skillet that had the onions. Sear for 3 – 4 minutes on each side. Pour the apple/onion mixture into a baking dish and top with the pork chops. Put the dish in the oven for 18 – 20 minutes. Mash the squash with a fork or masher. Serve a bottom layer of mashed squash, add a pork chop, and top with onion/apple mixture.

Yield: 1 serving

Ingredients

1 Tbsp olive oil
1/3 orange bell pepper, sliced
5 mushrooms, sliced
1 tsp crushed garlic
3 eggs, whisked

Directions:

Warm olive oil in a skillet and add bell pepper, mushrooms and garlic. Sauté for 5 - 7 minutes. Place in a bowl and set aside. Add the eggs to pan over medium heat. Cook thoroughly and add mixture over half of the omelet. Fold over and plate the omelet.

SHRIMP AND AVOCADO SALAD - LUNCH DAY 26

Yield: 2 servings

Ingredients

1 lb raw shrimp, peeled and
deveined
2 avocados, mashed
1 small red onion, minced
2 Tbsp olive oil
1 Tbsp hot sauce of choice
Juice of 1 lime
Juice of 1 lemon
1 garlic clove, minced
1/2 Tbsp garlic powder
1/2 cup cilantro
Salt to taste

Directions:

Preheat oven to 350°F. Toss shrimp in a bowl with olive oil. Lay shrimp on a lined baking sheet and sprinkle with salt and garlic powder. Bake for 15 minutes. In a bowl, mix together the avocado, hot sauce, lemon and lime juice, minced garlic, onion, cilantro and salt to taste. Serve the cooked shrimp with the avocado mash.

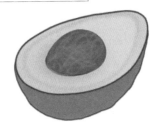

ARTICHOKE CHICKEN WITH CAPERS - DINNER DAY 26

Yield: 4 servings

Ingredients

4 Tbsp olive oil
1/4 onion, sliced
2 cups artichoke hearts, rinsed
1/4 cup capers, drained
Juice of 2 lemons
2 lbs chicken, bone-in

Directions:

Preheat oven to 375°F. Warm 2 Tbsp oil in a large skillet over medium heat. Sauté onions in the skillet until tender and add artichoke hearts, capers and lemon juice in the same pan and stir. Add the chicken pieces and remaining olive oil to the skillet and bake for 45 minutes.

EGGS YOUR WAY WITH APPLE CHICKEN PATTIES
BREAKFAST DAY 27

Yield: 4 servings

Ingredients

3 Tbsp coconut oil
1 lb ground chicken
1 apple, peeled and diced
2 Tbsp dried thyme
3 Tbsp dried parsley
2 Tbsp dried oregano
2 tsp garlic powder
Salt and pepper to taste
8 eggs

Directions

Preheat oven to 425°F. Warm coconut oil in pan over medium high heat and add apples, thyme, parsley and oregano about 7 – 8 minutes, or until apples are soft. Remove from heat and allow to cool for about 5 minutes. Combine the chicken with the contents of the skillet and mix well. Season with garlic powder, salt and pepper. Using your hands, form 12 patties from the meat mixture, about 1/2 " thick. Place the patties on a baking sheet lined with foil and bake for 20 minutes, or until internal temperature of the patties are 170°F. Serve with eggs cooked your favorite way!

GRILLED CHICKEN AND PINEAPPLE SKEWERS
LUNCH DAY 27

Yield: 3 servings

Ingredients

4 cups pineapple, cubed
1/4 cup olive oil
3 garlic cloves, minced
1 Tbsp ginger, minced
Juice of 1 lemon
1 tsp salt
1 Tbsp cilantro, minced
3 chicken breasts, cubed
Metal skewers

Directions:

Mix 1 cup pineapple, olive oil, garlic, ginger, lemon juice and salt in a bowl. Pour mixture into a blender or food processor and puree. Put mixture back in the bowl and add the minced cilantro, then set aside. Preheat the grill to medium high heat. Put the remaining pineapple and chicken chunks on your skewers and grill for 12 – 15 minutes. Turn the skewers every 4 - 5 minutes and brush with pineapple glaze several times while grilling.

SHREDDED BEEF WITH SWEET POTATO PLANKS
DINNER DAY 27

Yield: 4 – 6 servings

Ingredients

2 – 3 lb sirloin steak
2 large sweet potatoes
1 large yellow onion, sliced
1/2 cup beef broth
3 Tbsp olive oil
1 1/2 tsp salt, divided
1 tsp garlic powder
1 garlic clove, minced
1/2 tsp paprika
3/4 tsp black pepper, divided
1/4 tsp white pepper
1/4 tsp chili powder
1 Tbsp fresh thyme

Directions:

Put meat, onions and broth in a slow cooker. Season with 1 tsp salt, garlic powder, paprika, 1/4 tsp black pepper, white pepper and chili powder. Cook on low for 8 – 10 hours. Preheat oven to 350°F. Peel the sweet potatoes and cut into planks, approximately 1/2" thick. Mix together the olive oil, thyme, garlic, salt and pepper. Put the planks in the bowl and stir until coated with the mixture. Lay the sweet potatoes on a nonstick baking sheet in a single layer. Bake for 30 minutes, or until the potatoes start to brown on the edges. Once finished, shred the beef and serve on top of the sweet potato planks.

SAUSAGE SCOTCH EGGS - BREAKFAST DAY 28

Yield: 3 servings

Ingredients

6 medium hard-boiled eggs
1 lb breakfast sausage
1 1/2 tsp salt
1/2 tsp black pepper

Directions:

Preheat oven to 350°F. Mix sausage, salt and pepper in a bowl. Take 1/3 measuring cup and fill with mixture. Remove the mixture and flatten it with your hand to look like a hamburger patty, repeating until you have 6 patties. Place a peeled, hard-boiled egg in the center of each patty and fold around the whole egg, making sure the egg is sealed. Put eggs on a lined baking sheet and bake for 15 – 20 minutes.

Yield: 5 servings

Ingredients

5 boneless, skinless chicken breasts
1 large onion, chopped
3 qts chicken stock
2 cups celery, chopped
1 cup baby carrots
2 Tbsp gallons garlic powder
Dill weed to taste
Pepper to taste

Directions:

Put the rinsed chicken breast, chicken broth, onion, garlic powder, pepper and dill weed into a large soup pot. Cook over medium heat until soup boils. Reduce heat, cover and simmer for 30 minutes. Add the celery and carrots and continue cooking for one more hour. Shred the chicken before serving.

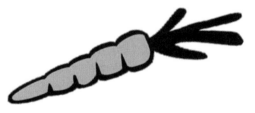

Yield: 2 servings

Ingredients

2 dozen large raw shrimp
4 zucchini or yellow squash
1/2 cup macadamia nuts
1 bunch cilantro, rinsed
1 clove garlic
1/2 cup olive oil
Salt and pepper to taste

Directions:

Make your pesto by pureeing the nuts, cilantro, garlic, oil, salt and pepper in a food processor until smooth. Peel and devein the raw shrimp. Make noodles by using a julienne peeler or spiralizer on the squash. Bring about an inch of water to a boil and place the noodles in a steamer basket for 3 – 5 minutes, then set aside. Steam the shrimp for about 3 minutes, or until pink all the way through. Combine the cooked noodles with the pesto until thoroughly mixed. Serve warm shrimp on top of the noodles.

Yield: 1 serving

Ingredients

1 Tbsp + 1 tsp coconut oil
2 cloves garlic, minced
1 orange bell pepper, chopped
1/2 onion, chopped
1 fresh jalapeno, minced
2 roma tomatoes, diced
2 eggs, whisked
Cilantro, for garnish
Avocado slices, for garnish
Salsa, for garnish

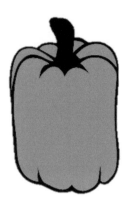

Directions:

In a medium skillet, warm 1 Tbsp coconut oil over medium heat and sauté the garlic, bell pepper, onion and jalapeno for 3 minutes. Add the tomato and sauté for 5 additional minutes, then set the pan aside. Warm 1 tsp coconut oil over medium low heat in a nonstick pan and scramble the eggs about 6 minutes, or until done. Plate the eggs next to the pepper and onion mixture and garnish with cilantro, avocado and salsa.

Yield: 1 serving

Ingredients

1 tsp coconut oil
1/2 yellow onion, diced
1/2 lb sausage, sliced
4 cups spinach

Directions:

Warm coconut oil over medium heat in a skillet and sauté onions until translucent. Add sausage and cook until brown, stirring occasionally. Add spinach and cover, reducing heat to low for about 5 minutes.

COD TACOS - DINNER DAY 29

Yield: 2 – 4 servings

Ingredients

1 – 2 pound cod filets
Juice from 1 lime
1 Tbsp olive oil
1/2 tsp chipotle powder
1 1/2 tsp ground cumin
1/2 tsp salt
Large lettuce leaves
2 cups shredded cabbage
1 cup mango, diced
1 1/2 cups jicama, peeled and
    diced
1 fresh jalapeno, minced
1/4 cup paleo mayonnaise
3/4 cup cilantro
Wedges from 1 lime

Directions:

Make a marinade by whisking together lime juice, olive oil, 1/4 tsp chipotle powder, 1 tsp cumin and salt. Let the fish rest in the marinade for 15 minutes. Make a slaw by mixing cabbage, mango, 1/2 cup diced cilantro, jicama, jalapeno, mayonnaise, 1/8 tsp chipotle powder and 1/2 tsp cumin. Warm a large pan to medium heat and add the fish and marinade. Cook each side for 3 – 4 minutes, or until the fish easily flakes. Take the skillet off the heat and flake the fish filets with a spatula. Plate with a large lettuce leaf filled with fish flakes, topped with slaw, and garnished with cilantro and lime juice.

HAM OMELET - BREAKFAST DAY 30

Yield: 1 serving

Ingredients

2 eggs
2 tsp coconut oil
1 Tbsp rosemary, chopped
1 Tbsp thyme, chopped
1/4 cup sliced ham
Salt and pepper to taste

Directions:

Mix eggs in a bowl. Warm coconut oil in a nonstick pan over medium heat and add eggs. Add rosemary, thyme, salt and pepper. Add ham to the center of the eggs after 1 – 2 minutes. Gently fold the sides in toward the middle once the edges are beginning to cook, and continue cooking until satisfied with the firmness of the omelet.

BRUSSELS SPROUT SALAD - LUNCH DAY 30

Yield: 2 servings

Ingredients

3 strips thick cut bacon
1 lb Brussels sprouts
1/3 cup blueberries
1/4 cup chopped walnuts
3 Tbsp lemon juice
1 garlic clove, minced
1/2 tsp dried tarragon
1/4 tsp dried mustard
1/4 tsp salt
1/8 tsp black pepper
1/4 cup olive oil

Directions:

Preheat the oven to 350°F. Place the bacon on a foil-lined baking sheet and bake for 15 – 20 minutes, or until crispy. Allow bacon to cool and chop into small pieces. Clean and slice the Brussels sprouts into thin pieces – approximately 4 – 6 per sprout. Put the slices in a large bowl with the blueberries and walnuts. In a smaller bowl, mix together lemon juice, garlic, tarragon, mustard, salt and pepper. Add the oil and continue mixing until the contents are combined. Toss the dressing in the salad and top with bacon.

BEEF AND BROCCOLI STIR FRY - DINNER DAY 30

Yield: 2 servings

Ingredients

2 Tbsp sesame oil
5 garlic cloves, minced
2 Tbsp ginger, minced
1 lb beef, cut into 1" cubes
4 cups broccoli florets
1/4 cup green onion, thinly
  sliced
1/4 cup coconut aminos
1 tsp each salt and pepper
1 tsp red pepper flakes

Directions:

Warm the sesame oil over high heat in a wok or pan. Sauté the ginger and garlic in the oil for 2 minutes, then add the steak. Stir and cook until the cubes are browned and seared. Mix in the broccoli, onion, coconut aminos, salt, pepper and red pepper flakes for an additional 2 – 3 minutes. Remove from pan and serve hot.

Snack Ideas

That's right, we're going to talk about snacks. Usually while talking about food or changing your eating habits, you expect to restrict yourself. Not this time! The anti-inflammatory challenge is not about weight loss, even though that may be a wonderful side effect. Instead, the challenge is about keeping your body healthy and happy.

Anything that is on our allowable foods list may be consumed as a snack. A few other ideas include:

❖ Raw nuts with dried or fresh fruit
❖ Apple slices or celery sticks with almond butter
❖ Sweet potato chips
❖ Pumpkin seeds
❖ Larabars (date/nut bars)
❖ Turkey slices with avocado

❖ Strawberry Banana Popsicles

Ingredients
    1 large banana, frozen
    12 strawberries
    1/2 cup almond milk

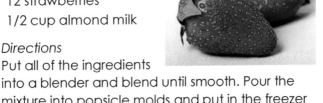

Directions
Put all of the ingredients into a blender and blend until smooth. Pour the mixture into popsicle molds and put in the freezer until frozen (about 8 hours). If your popsicle molds do not have a slot for sticks, add popsicle sticks in the middle after they have been in the freezer for 2 hours.

❖ Homemade fruit roll ups

Ingredients

    2 cups of your favorite berry

    6 mint leaves

    1/4 cup honey

Directions

Preheat the oven to 170°F. Put all of the ingredients into a blender and blend until smooth. Pour the mixture onto a baking sheet lined with parchment paper and spread evenly. Bake for 5 – 6 hours. Remove from the oven and allow to cool for at least 30 minutes. Cut into long strips and roll each strip.

Appetizer and Party Ideas

Going to parties and events can be one of the most difficult parts of following any type of diet. Let's face it, we live in a society where we can't seem to socialize without food. So how do we still have fun at parties without feeling deprived? We bring our own appetizers! Crazy thought, I know. Luckily there are thousands of anti-inflammatory appetizer recipes out there. You may find some of them more practical than others, and many of them are a hit with any crowd. Here are a few go-to appetizers from the team at Vitality Consultants.

Bacon or Turkey-Wrapped Asparagus

Ingredients

> 20 stalks of asparagus
> 10 pieces of bacon or sliced turkey

Directions

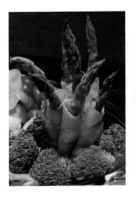

Preheat oven to 400°F. Clean and cut the bottom 2 inches off the asparagus. Cut the bacon or turkey in half and wrap each half around the asparagus stalk. Bake for 10 (if using turkey) or 25 (if using bacon) minutes. Serve warm.

Cauliflower Hummus

Ingredients

1 head cauliflower	4 tsp cumin
3/4 cup tahini	1 ½ tsp sea salt
1/4 cup olive oil	1 tsp paprika
3 Tbsp lemon juice	¼ tsp cayenne
5 cloves garlic	

Directions

Cut the cauliflower into small pieces and steam for about 6 minutes. While the cauliflower is steaming, run the tahini through a food processor for about 2 minutes. Smash the cloves of garlic with the side of a knife and place them in a skillet over medium heat for about 30 seconds, or until fragrant. Put the garlic into the food processor with the tahini and pulse until smooth. Add the steamed cauliflower to the food processor and run until the mixture looks like a sauce. Add the remaining ingredients and mix until well combined. Serve with veggies and enjoy!

Salmon Cucumber Planks

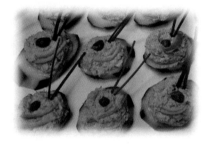

Ingredients

5 oz salmon
1/2 avocado
1 Tbsp lemon juice
1 Tbsp green onion, chopped
Salt and pepper to taste
1 large cucumber

Directions

Place salmon, avocado, lemon juice and green onion into a bowl and mash together. Mix in onion, salt and pepper. Cut cucumber into 1" slices and add salmon mixture to each slice.

In addition to these simple and delicious appetizers, try some staples such as:

- ❖ Sweet potato skins
- ❖ Fruit & veggie trays
- ❖ Mixed nuts
- ❖ Baked chicken wings
- ❖ Bacon-wrapped jalapeno poppers
- ❖ Gluten free turkey meatballs
- ❖ Boiled or steamed shrimp with homemade cocktail sauce

Just remember, don't let a gathering with friends ruin everything you have worked so hard for – have fun and eat smart!

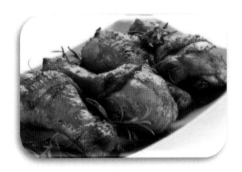

Weekly Menu Planner

	BREAKFAST	LUNCH	SNACK	DINNER
SUNDAY				
MONDAY				
TUESDAY				
WEDNESDAY				
THURSDAY				
FRIDAY				
SATURDAY				

Menu planning is one of the most beneficial things that you can do to set yourself up for success. If you plan all your meals in advance and buy groceries to make sure you have all of the necessary items, this lifestyle is much simpler. This template should be used as a guide to you after this challenge and the four week menu have come to an end.

To start, go through your calendar and figure out what you have planned for each day of the week. This prevents you from choosing a meal with a long preparation time even though it may not be realistic for that day. There are two ways to plan for days where you do not have time to cook. The first of which is to plan on using a slow cooker recipe. Our four week menu has a variety of slow cooker recipes including apple squash pork chops, shredded beef with sweet potato planks, turkey lasagna, squash and beef stew, Asian pork and spicy pulled pork. Most of these meals can be put into the slow cooker in the morning and enjoyed at dinnertime. The second option for busy days is to cook these meals ahead of time. For example, if on Tuesday morning you have a commitment that will prevent you from making lunch for the day, but Sunday night you have free time, you can use this time to cook your meal. Put the meal in a microwave safe container and reheat it for lunch.

Next, plan a rough sketch of what you would like to eat and be sure to include variety. For example, if you want a chicken dish on Wednesday for dinner, it may be wise to choose a recipe that contains beef for Thursday's lunch. This variety keeps you from getting bored or stuck in a rut with this anti-inflammatory challenge.

Fill in this template with the names of recipes, either from this challenge or an anti-inflammatory recipe you have found online or come up with on your own. Once your menu is planned, it is time to make a grocery list. Go through the ingredient lists for each recipe and determine what you already have in your kitchen. Bring your list of remaining ingredients to the grocery store and begin shopping. Be sure to stick to your list!

Tips:

- Shop on a day that is most convenient for you
- Start your weekly menu 1 - 2 days after this
- Have a go-to meal in your freezer for when life gets in the way and you need a quick meal when you are on the run

Guide to Organics

We know that purchasing organic foods all of the time can get expensive. But how do you know when it's okay to go conventional and when organic could be the better choice? Thankfully, there is an answer!

In 2013 the United States Department of Agriculture (USDA) took samples of over 3,000 pieces of produce. The laboratory results found over 165 pesticides on more than 1,000 of these samples. (Yikes!)

That's when the Environmental Working Group put together two lists of fruits and vegetables. The first list is called the Dirty Dozen™ and features the produce items that contained the highest amount of pesticides. These foods should be purchased organically whenever possible. In 2018, this list includes:

- ❖ Apples
- ❖ Celery
- ❖ Cherry tomatoes
- ❖ Cucumbers
- ❖ Grapes
- ❖ Nectarines
- ❖ Peaches
- ❖ Potatoes
- ❖ Snap peas
- ❖ Spinach
- ❖ Strawberries
- ❖ Sweet bell peppers

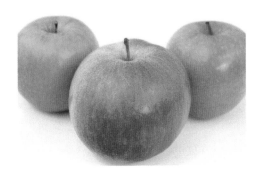

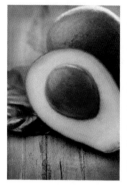

The second list of produce is called the Clean Fifteen™ and contains items that had the lowest amount of pesticides. Since these foods contain trace amounts of pesticides, they are considered safe to be eaten without the organic certification. This list includes:

- Avocados
- Cabbage
- Cantaloupe
- Cauliflower
- Eggplant
- Sweet peas
- Grapefruit

- Kiwis
- Mangoes
- Onions
- Papayas
- Pineapples
- Sweet corn
- Sweet potatoes

*This list is updated every year and produced by The Environmental Working Group.

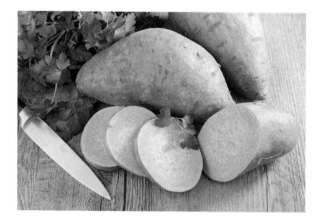

What Are Genetically Modified Organisms (GMOs)?

Large food industries have a lot of pressure on their shoulders. As a society, we expect food that stays fresh for weeks in our local stores year round. On their own, chickens do not grow fast enough, vegetables are not large enough, and fruit does not stay ripe long enough for these companies to keep up with the high standards of consumers nation-wide.

This is where modern biotechnology comes into play. Farmers can now create food that has all of the same characteristics that are demanded by society. This enhancement, or modification, of foods started almost 50 years ago when scientists learned that certain DNA traits can affect the quality of plants and animals. Biotechnology has advanced so far that scientists can now isolate a specific gene and replicate it to produce a more desirable product.

This can be great for farmers in terms of cost for a few reasons. First, it is easier to sell a seemingly perfect piece of produce. Second, some crops can be engineered so that they can protect themselves from damage done by insects, viruses and other diseases. Because these plants are defending themselves, farmers can often get by with using less insecticide. Not only are they reducing cost from using fewer chemicals, but less produce is being lost from spoilage. Third, scientists have even found a way to make some crops weather resistant. This extends the growing season, allowing farmers to generate income during the off-season.

In the United States, there are several agencies that oversee the safety of GMOs. The Food and Drug Administration makes sure that the food is safe for us to eat, the Environmental Protection Agency ensures that the pest control methods used are safe for human consumption and the United States Department of Agriculture makes sure that the fields the crops are growing in are safe. Unfortunately, the research and tests used to ensure the safety of GMOs are paid for and administered by the manufacturers that produced the seeds. Skeptics believe this may lead to questionable integrity on behalf of these studies. In fact, over 60 countries around the world have restricted or banned the use of GMOs in their farming practices, which makes the tests done in the U.S. appear even more questionable.

Sadly, the government does not require foods that are genetically modified to be labeled. This means that there is truly no way to know which foods have been affected by modern biotechnology and which haven't. If you are looking to stay away from GMOs, it is best to purchase from a local farmer or look for foods labeled non-GMO. Make sure to ask farmers questions about how their food is grown!

Why No Beans and Legumes

If you don't like beans, you're in luck! They are not part of the anti-inflammatory challenge. If you're a bean fanatic, continue reading to understand why they are not recommended under anti-inflammatory guidelines. Looking at their nutrient content, you will find that they are typically high in protein, low in fat and high in fiber. Unfortunately, the nutrition information is deceiving in regard to how beans and legumes affect the body.

For starters, beans and legumes contain phytic acid. Phytic acid binds to nutrients in the food, which prevents the body from absorbing them. So while they may contain many desirable nutrients, your body may never get to utilize them.

Beans and legumes are a high FODMAP[2] food. Food that falls into this category tends to cause digestive issues, especially if you have a pre-existing condition, including irritable bowel syndrome, colitis and Crohn's disease. Symptoms that may occur include abdominal pain, bloating and changes in bowel habits.

Beans and legumes also contain a type of protein called lectins. These proteins are created by plants to ward off predators. Lectins are found in a wide variety of foods, but the amount and type of lectins present in the food may cause problems. People react to different lectins in different ways. Lectins are found to be most harmful in grains, legumes and dairy. The proteins found

---

[2] FODMAP stands for fermentable, oligosaccharides, disaccharides, monosaccharides and polyols

in these items have been known to damage the intestinal wall and may cause leaky gut syndrome, which is associated with many other digestive and autoimmune disorders.

Here is a list of common beans and legumes that are best avoided:

- Alfalfa
- Black beans
- Black-eyed peas
- Chickpeas
- Chili beans
- Kidney beans
- Licorice

- Lima beans
- Navy beans
- Peas
- Peanuts
- Pinto beans
- Red beans
- Soy beans

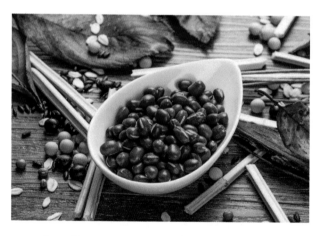

There are two items on this list that have even further health implications than the ones previously stated.

Peanuts: Peanuts are a sneaky type of legume. They contain the other properties of beans and legumes that were mentioned earlier, but also contain a mold called aflatoxin. This mold is what causes many people to be allergic to peanuts. Even for those who are not allergic to aflatoxins, the body may recognize it as an invader and cause an inflammatory response.

Soy: Soy is another legume that disguises itself as healthy. After all, tofu and soy milk can't be that bad for you, right? Unfortunately, this is wrong. Along with phytic acid, FODMAPs and lectins, soy also contains phytoestrogens. Phytoestrogen imitates estrogen in the body, making the body believe that it has enough of the hormone. The issue with this is that the phytoestrogens do not perform any of the functions that estrogen does. This hormone imbalance can lead to further health problems in both men and women.

Because of all the negative health issues that can occur due to beans and legumes, they are eliminated from an anti-inflammatory diet.

Why No Grains

For many people, grains are the most difficult thing to give up when changing eating habits. Right now, I'm sure it seems unimaginable to go for 30 days without bread, cereal and pasta. As discussed during the "what to expect during the first 30 days" section, during the first two weeks you may experience some cravings for the old staples in your diet. This is normal. Don't give into these cravings though! After your 30 days is up you'll forget why they were such an important part of your diet in the first place.

First things first, let's talk about gluten. Unless you've been living in a hole for the past few years, you've likely heard about the "gluten-free craze." What you may not know is that this fad has some science behind it (crazy, I know). Gluten is a protein found in barley, rye and wheat that is a combination of two proteins called gliadin and glutenin.[3]

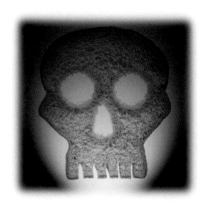 Gluten is difficult for the body to fully digest. When food goes through the gastrointestinal (GI) tract undigested, the intestinal cells attack the particle as if it were a foreign invader. The impact of this attack is individual, but can range from mild intestinal inflammation to severe

---

[3] Some oats contain gluten, not by nature, but due to the process in which they are made. Corn and corn starch contain gliadin, one of the components of gluten.

damage to the GI tract that prevents absorption of other food. Removing gluten from the diet can prevent and ease this damage. The addition of anti-inflammatory foods can help further reduce and potentially eliminate inflammation. There are certainly gluten free substitutes, but many of these products are filled with added fats and sugars to make up for the texture lost by leaving out gluten. My suggestion is to try substituting gluten-containing foods with whole foods. For example, zucchini makes great noodles in a dish that was originally pasta-based, lettuce can replace a tortilla or bread and make a delicious wrap, and cauliflower easily transforms into bread or pizza crust.

While gluten is found in most grains, there are certainly some that are gluten free including rice, quinoa and buckwheat. Unfortunately, these are not recommended under an anti-inflammatory diet either. Refined grains, such as white rice, are also discouraged. They are high in carbohydrates, and the refining process strips them of many nutrients that were originally present. While the whole grain versions are better for you (they contain some nutrients along with fiber to slow down digestion), they have some inflammatory properties. Like beans, grains contain toxic lectins that disrupt digestion. Though each person has an individual response to these toxins, the most common side effect is the protein passing through the intestinal wall and entering the blood stream. The response to this is similar to that of gluten. The body sees the particle as an invader and attacks it, leading to inflammation.

To avoid inflammation, it is best to avoid all grains. There are many ways to replace grains with whole foods, and I encourage you to find a few favorites during this challenge.

What's the Deal with Refined Sugar, Artificial Sweeteners and Natural Sweeteners?

The use of refined sugars, refined/artificial sweeteners and natural sweeteners appears to be a topic that has been confusing people for centuries. Many people are unsure of their views regarding these substances, or where they fit into their diet. Continue reading for a brief description of each type of sweetener and to determine where they fit in an anti-inflammatory lifestyle.

Refined Sugar

Refined sugar, or table sugar, is created by (surprise!) refining a sugar cane plant. The refining process involves cutting up and washing the sugar cane and extracting its juice. This juice is then thickened, bleached and mixed with a variety of chemicals. This thickened mixture is boiled until it turns into a crystallized paste. The crystallized sugar is removed from the liquid portion and is washed and dehydrated, forming the sugar molecules that we are familiar with.

Added sugar in baked goods and beverages are not the only places that we find refined sugar. Simple carbohydrates, found in white breads and pasta, are broken down into sugar in the body and processed the same way.

Because of the intense refining process and effect that refined sugar has on the body, it is not recommended as a part of an anti-inflammatory diet.

Artificial Sweeteners

Artificial sweeteners are additives that taste sweeter than sugar, but provide few or no calories. There are six artificial sweeteners approved for use in the United States, but only three are widely used. Continue reading for a description of aspartame, saccharin, and sucralose.

1) *Aspartame*: Aspartame, the key ingredient in Equal, NutraSweet and NutraTaste, is 200 times sweeter than table sugar. It was invented in 1965 when a scientist was researching a treatment for ulcers. According to Dr. Joseph Mercola, aspartame was approved by the FDA, "not on scientific grounds, but rather because of strong political and financial pressure." In fact, the FDA began a criminal investigation on the research about aspartame due to concealed and misrepresented research facts. After much debate and political turnover, aspartame was approved for use in dry products in 1981 and liquids in 1983. Use of aspartame is linked to fibromyalgia, migraines and diabetes. Though there have been over 10,000 complaints about the additive made to the FDA, aspartame is found in over 6,000 foods.

2) *Saccharin*: Saccharin, also known as Sweet'N Low, is 500 times sweeter than table sugar. It was invented in 1879 by a scientist researching toluene derivatives. (Toluene is a clear liquid that smells similar to paint thinners). In 1912, saccharin was banned from the United States because of potential health risks associated with its intake.

The ban was lifted during World War I due to sugar shortages resulting in an increased need of artificial sweeteners. Even though saccharin was removed from the FDA's Generally Recognized as Safe (GRAS) list, it is still widely used today.

3) *Sucralose*: Sucralose, commonly known as Splenda, is 600 times sweeter than table sugar. It was invented in 1976 when scientists were trying to create an insecticide. Sucralose was denied FDA approval for twelve years, before being approved for use in 1998. Splenda, a brand name for sucralose, has a slogan that says it is "made from sugar so it tastes like sugar." Sucralose is made by taking sugar, and treating it with twelve different molecules. (Yikes!)

Artificial sweeteners have been linked to many inflammatory diseases, especially for those who are prone to inflammation. Because of this and the chemical makeup of many artificial sweeteners, they are not a recommended part of an anti-inflammatory diet.

Natural Sweeteners

Of the sweet products listed here, natural sweeteners are the best option and are allowable under anti-inflammatory guidelines. Natural sweeteners are found in nature and do not undergo a refining process before being consumed. Because they are not refined, these sweeteners are easier for the body to break down, reducing the risk of inflammation that occurs. Natural sugars should be consumed in moderation, as they can cause blood sugar levels to rise. If your blood sugar rises too high or too quickly, inflammation may occur.

Our favorite natural sweeteners are stevia, honey and maple syrup. Continue reading for a brief description of each.

1. *Stevia:* Stevia is 150 times sweeter than refined sugar and comes from the stevia plant. There are many forms of stevia, and not all brands are created equal. Look for stevia products with few additives.

   ❖ The stevia leaf is the most natural form of stevia available. You can chew the leaf to extract sweetness or dry the leaf and powder it.

   ❖ Stevia can also be purchased in a liquid form. The liquid is created by boiling the leaves in water to extract the sweetness. These products are made by adding natural flavors and oils to the boiled stevia leaf.

   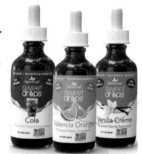

   ❖ Powdered stevia is the most processed form of stevia and is made by drying the plant's leaves and putting them through a crystallization process to form a powder.

Stevia Conversion Chart

Amount of Sugar	Powdered Stevia Equivalent	Liquid Stevia Equivalent
1 teaspoon	A pinch	2 – 4 drops
1 tablespoon	¼ teaspoon	6 – 9 drops
1 cup	1 teaspoon	1 teaspoon

2. *Honey:* Honey is an anti-inflammatory food. When consumed, a protein in the nectar of bees

suppresses inflammation in the body. Honey has a low glycemic index, meaning that it is absorbed slower in the body and does not cause blood sugar levels to rise quickly. Along with water and sugar, honey contains a variety of B vitamins, calcium, copper, iron, magnesium, manganese, phosphorus, potassium, sodium and zinc.

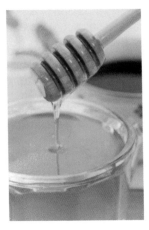

- ❖ When substituting honey for sugar in recipes, use 2/3 cup to 3/4 cup of honey for every cup of sugar.
- ❖ Decrease your oven temperature by 25 degrees. Honey makes your food brown faster.
- ❖ For each cup of honey used, decrease the amount of liquid in the recipe by 1/4 cup.

3. *Pure maple syrup:* Maple syrup has over 54 compounds that are beneficial for our health. It was found that many of these components contain both anti-inflammatory and antioxidant properties.
    - ❖ Maple syrup is a great option for sweetening applesauce, chicken, granola, oatmeal, yogurt and much more.
    - ❖ When substituting maple syrup for sugar in recipes, use 3/4 cup of maple syrup for every cup of sugar.
    - ❖ For each cup of maple syrup used, decrease the amount of liquid in the recipe by 3 tablespoons.

Does Fat Make You Fat?

Fat has had a pretty bad reputation. We seem to spend most of our lives trying to lose fat or trying not to get fat, so why eat it?

Fat has many roles in the body. It supports immune function, blood clotting, muscle contractions and blood pressure. Fat helps insulate the body, promote brain function and lubricates some of the body surfaces. I bet you didn't know fat was needed for all of that! Fat also helps some vitamins, known as fat-soluble vitamins, to be utilized by the body. These vitamins include vitamins A, D, E and K.

Hopefully it is clear that fat is not the bad guy – and is even a necessary part of your diet. So why don't we eat *more* fat? Eating the wrong types of fat, or too much of the good types, can promote inflammation in the body and lead to chronic disease.

Before we discuss the different types of fats, there are a few terms that you should be familiar with.

- ❖ *HDL cholesterol*: known as the "good" cholesterol, carries blood cholesterol away from blood vessels and into the liver to be excreted.
- ❖ *LDL cholesterol*: known as the "bad" cholesterol, carries cholesterol to the body to be used. LDL cholesterol can deposit cholesterol onto artery walls (this causes a buildup of plaque).
- ❖ *Triglycerides:* a form of fat that is found in both the body and food. Triglycerides cause the liver to make more cholesterol, increasing the amount of LDL cholesterol in the blood.

There are four main types of fat – monounsaturated, polyunsaturated, saturated and trans. The table below describes each type, what food sources they can be found in and how they influence cholesterol in the body.

Type of Fat	Description	Sources	Effect
Monounsaturated	Usually liquid at room temperature and become a solid when chilled. Typically contain high amounts of vitamin E, an anti-oxidant.	Nuts, canola oil, olive oil, avocados, sunflower oil and seeds	↓ total cholesterol, ↓ LDL cholesterol, may ↑ HDL cholesterol
Polyunsaturated	Liquid at room temperature and remain liquid when chilled. Provide essential fatty acids that cannot be made in the body: omega-3 and omega-6 fatty acids.	Corn, safflower, soybean, sesame, and sunflower oils, walnuts, fatty fish (salmon, mackerel, herring, trout, sardines), and wheat germ	↓ total cholesterol, ↓ LDL cholesterol, ↓ HDL cholesterol
Saturated	Solid at room temperature, causing the fat to accumulate in artery walls. However, medium- and short-chain fatty acids, like the ones found in coconut oil, may boost immune function and promote gastrointestinal health. This is why coconut oil is allowed on an anti-inflammatory diet.	Animal-based foods (fatty meats, eggs, butter, whole milk, dairy made from whole milk), fried foods, fast food, and coconut and palm oils	↑ total cholesterol, ↑ LDL cholesterol
Trans	Man-made fats created by turning a liquid fat into a solid fat. This process is called hydrogenation. Once consumed, trans fat acts like saturated fat in the body.	Hydrogenated fats, margarine, shortening, microwave popcorn, and commercially made baked goods	↑ total cholesterol, ↑ LDL cholesterol, may ↓ HDL cholesterol

As we discussed, fat is necessary in the diet. However too much fat can be a bad thing, and saturated and trans fat can raise the "bad" cholesterol in your body. For these reasons, total fat should be limited to 20 - 30% of your daily calories in an anti-inflammatory diet. Saturated fat should make up less than 7% of your daily calories, and trans fat should be as limited as possible.

Omega-3 fatty acids should be consumed on a regular basis. These essential fatty acids help the body fight inflammation and reduce the risk of heart disease and stroke. Omega-3s also combat the inflammatory effects that occur after consuming omega-6 fatty acids.

Sources of omega-3 fatty acids include:

- ❖ Nut and fish oils
- ❖ Fatty fish
- ❖ Flaxseed
- ❖ Chia seeds
- ❖ Pumpkin seeds
- ❖ Hemp seeds

Sources of omega-6 fatty acids include:

- ❖ Walnuts
- ❖ Cashews
- ❖ Vegetable, soybean, canola oils
- ❖ Almonds
- ❖ Sunflower seeds

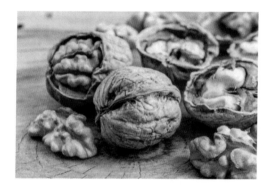

The typical American diet tends to be high in omega-6 fatty acids due to the common use of vegetable oils found in processed foods. In fact, the omega-3 to omega-6 ratio is typically 1:16 in most diets. When following the anti-inflammatory diet, the ratio that we are striving for is 1:1 meaning that the amount of omega-3 fatty acids is identical to the amount of omega-6 fatty acids in the diet.

Eggs –
To Yolk or Not To Yolk

You've likely heard that eggs are high in cholesterol and it is best to eat just the egg whites. It is very common to hear people say that they would like an egg white omelet, and eggs can even be purchased in containers without the yolk. With many conflicting thoughts about which part of the eggs are the best for you, we thought it was important to discuss both parts of the egg and how they fit into an anti-inflammatory diet.

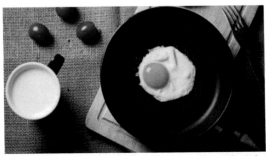

We can't begin a conversation about eggs without first talking about cholesterol. It must be noted that the cholesterol you consume in the diet (dietary cholesterol) is different than the cholesterol found in the blood (blood cholesterol). Excessive blood cholesterol is what can lead to an accumulation of plaque in the arteries and increase a person's risk for heart disease.

Dietary cholesterol usually comes from animal sources of food. Dietary cholesterol does not directly influence blood cholesterol. In fact, a diet high in saturated and trans fats is more likely to raise blood cholesterol than dietary cholesterol. The current recommendations for cholesterol consumption is to consume no more than 300 mg per day. One large egg contains about 190 mg.

Recent studies show that a person can eat about 7 eggs (including the yolk) a week with no spike in cholesterol. However, if you have diabetes or heart disease, you should check with your doctor to determine if eggs can be a part of your diet.

Now that we got the discussion about cholesterol out of the way, let's discuss the other nutrients that an egg has to offer. The egg yolk contains all of the vitamins A, D, E and K that are in an egg. The yolk also contains 90% of the calcium, choline, folate, iron, phosphate, thiamin, zinc and vitamins B6 and B12. The last benefit of the yolk is that it contains omega-3 fatty acids. If you only eat egg whites, you are missing out on these great nutrients, some of which have antioxidant properties.

Looking at the anti-inflammatory properties of an egg yolk, it seems obvious that it should be eaten. If you are advised to limit your cholesterol, it may be wise to limit yourself to no more than one egg yolk per day and using egg whites for the remainder of your meal.

Pros and Cons of Nuts

Nuts are a staple in an anti-inflammatory diet. They make great replacements for flour in baking, create a good alternative for peanut butter and make a great breading for meat. Nuts are a good addition to trail mix and granola and make great snacks.

Though all nuts are different, most are very nutrient dense. They are high in protein and have a variety of vitamins and minerals, including the antioxidant and anti-inflammatory vitamin E. They also have a respectable amount of calcium, which is important to those of us following an anti-inflammatory diet as we are cutting out dairy. Eating nuts can lower your "bad" cholesterol and decreases the risk of developing heart disease. Nuts are great sources of the anti-inflammatory fatty acid omega-3.

Though omega-3 fats are beneficial in reducing inflammation, too much of them can actually have adverse effects. Along with the high calorie content that comes along with a high fat diet, eating too much can increase the likelihood of developing a chronic disease. This is why nuts should be consumed in moderation; a small handful is the perfect amount.

Another concern with nuts is that they are typically eaten raw, and there is a chance that there may be harmful bacteria on the surface. To be safe either purchase organic nuts or roast them before eating.

Check out this trail mix recipe to incorporate nuts as a delicious snack!

Trail Mix

Ingredients:

  1 cup raw cashews
  1 cup raw almonds
  1 cup raw pumpkin seeds
  1 ½ tsp ground cinnamon
  Pinch nutmeg
  Pinch cayenne pepper
  2 Tbsp pure maple syrup
  ½ cup unsweetened coconut flakes

Directions:

Preheat the oven to 400°F and line a rimmed baking sheet with parchment paper. In a large bowl, mix all ingredients until well combined. Spread mixture onto the baking sheet in an even layer and bake for 8 minutes, mixing after 4 minutes. Let cool and serve at room temperature.

Guide to Reading Labels

Following an anti-inflammatory diet requires extra attention to be put on what is in the foods we are eating. This is easy when it comes to fresh food, but most of the food found in American culture is packaged. To determine if packaged food is anti-inflammatory, we turn to the food label. Unfortunately, the label often leads to confusion.

So what is on the label? By law, each food label must contain some specific information including the name of the product, name and address of the manufacturer, amount of product in the container, ingredients, Nutrition Facts, and common allergens. There are specific nutrients that must appear on the Nutrition Facts label including fat, saturated fat, trans fat, cholesterol, sodium, total carbohydrates, dietary fiber, sugar, protein, vitamins A and C, calcium and iron. Other nutrients may be added, but they are not required.[4]

Nutrition Facts

Serving Size 1 bar (24g)
Servings Per Container 10

Amount Per Serving

Calories 100   Calories from Fat 25

	% Daily Value*
Total Fat 2.5g	4%
Saturated Fat 1g	5%
Trans Fat 0g	
Polyunsaturated Fat 0g	
Monounsaturated Fat 1g	
Cholesterol 0mg	0%
Sodium 80mg	3%
Potassium 60mg	2%
Total Carbohydrate 18g	6%
Dietary Fiber 1g	4%
Sugars 7g	
Protein 2g	

Vitamin A 0%	•	Vitamin C 0%
Calcium 8%	•	Iron 4%

*Percent Daily Values are based on a 2,000 calorie diet. Your daily values may be higher or lower depending on your calorie needs:

	Calories	2,000	2,500
Total Fat	Less than	65g	80g
Sat Fat	Less than	20g	25g
Cholesterol	Less than	300mg	300mg
Sodium	Less than	2,400mg	2,400mg
Potassium		3,500mg	3,500mg
Total Carbohydrate		300g	375g
Dietary Fiber		25g	30g

INGREDIENTS: GRANOLA (WHOLE GRAIN ROLLED OATS, WHOLE GRAIN BROWN RICE FLOUR, SUGAR, WHOLE WHEAT FLAKES, HIGH OLEIC CANOLA OIL, MOLASSES, ENRICHED WHEAT FLOUR [BLEACHED WHEAT FLOUR, MALTED BARLEY FLOUR, NIACIN, REDUCED IRON, THIAMIN MONONITRATE, RIBOFLAVIN, FOLIC ACID], CALCIUM CARBONATE, SODIUM BICARBONATE, NONFAT DRY MILK, SOY LECITHIN, CARAMEL COLOR), WHOLE GRAIN BROWN RICE FLOUR, CORN SYRUP, INVERT SUGAR, SEMISWEET CHOCOLATE CHIPS (SUGAR, CHOCOLATE LIQUOR, COCOA BUTTER, SOY LECITHIN, SALT, VANILLA), PEANUT BUTTER FLAVORED CHIPS (SUGAR, PARTIALLY DEFATTED PEANUT FLOUR, PALM KERNEL AND PALM OIL, NONFAT DRY MILK, DEXTROSE, SOY LECITHIN, SALT), PEANUT BUTTER (ROASTED PEANUTS), CORN SYRUP SOLIDS, GLYCERIN, LESS THAN 2% OF: SUGAR, PEANUT OIL, CALCIUM CARBONATE, SALT, MOLASSES, HONEY, NATURAL AND ARTIFICIAL FLAVORS, CITRIC ACID, CARAMEL COLOR, MIXED TOCOPHEROLS (A PRESERVATIVE).

CONTAINS WHEAT, MILK, SOY AND PEANUT.

DISTRIBUTED BY SUPERVALU INC. EDEN PRAIRIE, MN 55344 USA

The first thing that I urge you to look at is the allergen warnings on the label. This is the simplest way to eliminate some foods that cause inflammation. Be

---

[4] An exception to this rule is labels that have a nutrient content claim. For example, if a label says that a food is a "good source of vitamin K," vitamin K must be present on the Nutrition Facts.

on the lookout for foods containing milk, peanuts, wheat and soybeans (in addition to any other allergens you may be sensitive to). As an example, let's look at the food label to the left. Without looking at any of the ingredients or nutrition information, we can easily see that this food is not acceptable under anti-inflammatory guidelines. The label clearly states that the item contains wheat, milk, soy and peanuts – all things that are not recommended. That was easy.

Next, take a look at the ingredient list. Typically, the fewer ingredients the better. Be sure to read through all the ingredients and be sure that the item does not contain gluten or grains, corn, dairy, refined sugar or high fructose corn syrup, or legumes (including soy and peanuts). Refined sugar is one of the most difficult things to spot in the ingredient list, because it has many forms that fall under different names. In general, words that end in –ose (such as dextrose and maltose) are a form of sugar. In addition to the –ose forms, stay away from the following types of sugar:

- Brown sugar
- Cane sugar
- Confectioner's sugar
- Corn sweeteners
- Corn syrup
- Crystallized cane sugar
- Dextrin
- Erythritol
- Evaporated cane juice
- Fruit juice concentrate
- High-fructose corn syrup
- Hydrogenated starch hydrolysates
- Invert sugar
- Isomalt
- Lactitol
- Malt syrup
- Maltitol
- Mannitol
- Raw sugar
- Sorbitol
- Turbinado sugar
- Xylitol

Check for items that are sweetened with a natural sweetener, such as stevia, honey or maple syrup.

Depending on your doctor's recommendations, you may look at other things on the food label. If you are trying to lose weight, the serving size, calories and fat content will guide your decisions about which foods to buy. For those of you that are diabetic, you may need to count the total number of carbohydrates in an item. People with heart failure will likely be checking the amount of sodium in their food.

Your first few trips to the grocery store will likely be time consuming. Write down which brands meet anti-inflammatory guidelines and continue purchasing them. You may find that it is much easier to purchase whole foods and make your own snacks. Whichever you prefer, find a system that works for you and stick with it.

Tips on Freezable Foods

Freezing is a great way to preserve foods. However, it is important to follow proper storage techniques. After all, what is the point of following anti-inflammatory guidelines if you are going to get sick from eating spoiled foods? For best freezing practices, keep your freezer at or below 0°F.

When you purchase frozen foods at the grocery store, be sure to store them in their original packaging. They are usually sold in airtight packages which will prevent freezer burn. If you cannot use the original packaging because you cooked the food at home, use a container or bag that is meant to be stored in the freezer (check the packaging information on your Tupperware and zip-bags). Be sure to label these containers with a description of the food and the date they were put into freezer and use them within the recommended time. Use the chart provided as a guide for storage times.

Vegetables should be blanched prior to freezing. This allows them to have a longer freezer life. To blanch vegetables, put them into boiling water for about three minutes and

Food	Length of time in freezer
Deli-sliced meats	1-2 months
Fresh beef, veal, lamb, pork	
Steaks	6-12 months
Chops	4-6 months
Roasts	4-12 months
Fresh poultry	
Chicken or turkey, whole	9 months
Pieces	3-4 months
Fresh fish	
Lean fish	6 months
Fatty fish	2-3 months
Smoked fish	2 months in vacuum package
Shellfish	3-6 months
Ham and corned beef	
Ham, fully cooked	1-2 months
Corned beef	Drained, 1 month
Ground and stew meats	
Stew meats	3-4 months
Ground meats	3-4 months
Bacon and sausage	1-2 months
Soups and stews	2-3 months
Cooked meat or poultry	2-6 months

Source: Adapted from www.foodsafety.gov

immediately place them into cold water to stop them from further cooking. Freeze them in zippered plastic bags that are suitable for freezing.

Thawing foods is just as (if not more) important than freezing them. Foods should never be thawed on the counter because bacteria grows very quickly at room temperature. There are three safe ways to thaw food.

1. **In the refrigerator.** This takes planning! Food thawed in the refrigerator takes multiple hours, even a full day depending on the size and type of food. Take the item out of the freezer and put it on a plate to collect any liquid that will drip from it. Food that is thawed in the refrigerator can be kept for 1-3 days after cooking and should be cooked before refreezing.
2. **In the microwave:** If you do not have time to thaw food in the refrigerator, remove the packaging and put it in a microwave safe container. Food can safely be defrosted on the low or defrost settings. Food that is thawed in the microwave should be cooked immediately before eating or refreezing.
3. **In cold water.** Frozen meat, poultry or fish can be defrosted in cold water, as long as the water is changed every 30 minutes. The meat should be in a vacuum-sealed or zippered bag with no leaks. Food that is thawed in cold water should be cooked immediately before eating or refreezing.

Remember, food can be prepared without being thawed first, but it will take about 50% longer to cook than it would otherwise.

Let's Talk Cocktails

Don't worry, we're not here to tell you that you can no longer drink – that's just not how we do things. We do, however, ask that you follow a few simple guidelines.

Look for gluten-free choices

Most liquor goes through a distillation process that dilutes any gluten that was originally in the product to amounts so small that the Food and Drug Administration considers it safe for those with celiac disease, making them acceptable for an anti-inflammatory diet. Unfortunately, some (not all) people with celiac disease or gluten intolerance may experience gluten reactions when drinking vodka, whiskey or scotch. It is unknown exactly what causes these reactions, though many experts believe that trace amounts of gluten may be added back to the product after distillation for flavor. In any case, those with celiac disease or gluten intolerance are advised to drink small amounts of scotch, whiskey and vodka and determine if it causes a reaction. There are also liquors that are not manufactured using wheat including tequila, rum and potato vodka.

Wine – yum! Wine is made from grapes, which are gluten free. You have probably heard that it is recommended to have a glass of red wine every night. That is because red wine contains many antioxidant properties, which coincidentally protect against inflammation!

Are you a beer drinker? Don't worry, you don't have to give it up! At least look for gluten-free options. Heineken is available at most bars and many apple ciders are gluten-free. A brand of beer called Omission has begun brewing a variety of craft beers in which the gluten has been removed. Check the label of other beers to determine if they have the gluten removed.

Choose your mixers wisely

Sodas and sugary beverages are not allowed under an anti-inflammatory diet. Fortunately, we have come up with a number of solutions.

1. Choose low-calorie beverage that do not contain added sugars. Good options include unsweetened tea, 100% fruit juice and club soda. You can make your own lemon-lime soda by ordering a club soda and squeezing lemon and lime slices to taste. Purchase flavored water, but make sure that it doesn't have artificial sweeteners such as sucralose, aspartame or saccharin.

2. Use SweetLeaf Stevia products. Is a rum and coke your favorite drink? Simply make or order a rum and seltzer water, and add about 15 drops of cola flavored stevia. In the mood for a lemon drop? Order your favorite vodka and sparkling 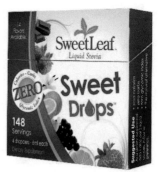 water and add one full dropper of lemon stevia. This is where your creativity can come into play! There are a wide selection of SweetLeaf flavors including:

- Apricot nectar
- Chocolate
- Coconut
- Cola
- English toffee
- Hazelnut
- Lemon
- Peppermint
- Peppermint mocha
- Pumpkin spice
- Root beer
- Stevia clear
- Valencia orange
- Vanilla crème

Whatever your drink choice, remember to not let your alcohol intake affect your food choices. Do you like to have a snack after a few cocktails? Be prepared! Pack snacks ahead of time. If you have a tendency to eat poorly the morning after a good time, have your breakfast pre-made so it is convenient, or make a double portion of it.

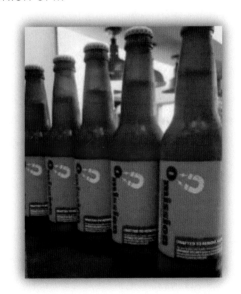

NOTE: If you are allergic to gluten check the label to ensure that your choice of alcohol and mixers was never cross-contaminated with any wheat products.

Tips on Making This Lifestyle Affordable

Being a registered dietitian, people constantly tell me that they can't follow any specific eating plan because it costs too much. What I want to say is "DO YOU KNOW HOW MUCH IT COSTS TO BE IN THE HOSPITAL AND TREATED FOR CHRONIC DISEASE?" The average cost of staying in a Missouri hospital is over $2,052 per day.[5] According to the Centers for Disease Control and Prevention, the average length of stay for a patient with a first time diagnosis of heart disease is 4.6 days. So by purchasing cheap, processed food instead of fresh produce and lean meat, you are spending over $8,700 for your *first* visit in the hospital. Not to mention the additional cost of any surgeries, follow-up appointments and medication that you are likely going to be prescribed.

But since that's not an "appropriate" or "professional" response, I help them come up with ways to make their prescribed diet more affordable. (I know, how boring.) Here are some tips that have certainly come in handy for me, and will hopefully help save you money as well!

Eating out

First thing's first, you're going to have to spend more time in your kitchen and less time eating out. Eating out is obviously enjoyable and brings friends together. However, it's well known that eating out does two things:

---

[5] Average cost in 2016, according to Becker's Hospital Review.

1) Encourages you to stray away from anti-inflammatory guidelines.
2) Costs so much more than cooking at home!

Eating out costs about $15 per person. But that's for normal people. You are no longer considered "normal". You will likely have to make substitutions to the menu items to make your meal anti-inflammatory. This can add an additional $2-5 to the final cost. And is it worth it? Not usually. You never know what types of oil and sauces are being added to your meal. You could be served a plate full of inflammation without even knowing it. To be safe, ask your server a lot of questions about the way your meals are prepared, learn to eat before heading out with friends, and dine out less frequently. To start, try cutting the number of times you eat out per month in half.

At the store

Be wise about where you are shopping and spend some time shopping around for the best prices. Do you not know how much coconut oil or dates typically cost? Spend a day going to about three grocery stores and compare the price of these items. Consider looking at how much food costs per ounce, which is often found on the price tag. Write down where each item is the cheapest and make sure to buy it at that store.

Another tip is to purchase food in bulk. Just make sure you are buying shelf stable items or food that you are certain you can eat before they go bad. After all, what's the point in saving $1.50 per ounce if you waste 6 ounces? Things that I recommend buying in bulk include oil, frozen meat and fish, flour and nuts.

If you live in a rural area and do your shopping at Walmart, download their app! There is a "Savings Catcher" inside the app. All you have to do is scan your receipt and Walmart spends about two days price-checking it for you. If there are items at other stores advertised for cheaper, Walmart puts the difference on the app. Once your account builds up money, you can spend it on anything you want in the store.

Farmer's market

Find a farmer's market near you and get to know the vendors. Aside from the food being fresh and in-season, food from the farmer's market is often much cheaper than food from the grocery store.

If you get to know the vendors or go to the market right before they close, you will likely get a discounted price. The vendors like to give cheaper prices to customers that they know will come back to them in the future, and at the end of the day their food will likely go to waste if unsold.

If you find a great deal on produce but know you will not be able to use it, buy it anyway! You can always freeze fresh fruit to eat raw or use in smoothies. Tomatoes can be made into salsa or spaghetti sauce and frozen in small batches to defrost later in the year.

Grow your own produce

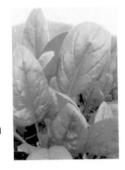

If you have some land in your yard, or even pots inside your house, you can start a garden! Growing your own fresh herbs, fruits or vegetables is a great way to save money. Look online to find out what type of produce grows best in each season.

Seeds or small plants can be bought from a hardware store or in the early weeks of a local farmer's market. They are relatively cheap, and if cared for properly produce a lot of crop. An added bonus? This can be a great way to get your children excited about eating vegetables or seasoning their food!

DIY

Have you ever looked on Google or Pinterest for "anti-inflammatory sauces?" You can find thousands of recipes for homemade ketchup, salad dressing, BBQ sauce, hummus, mayonnaise and more. Not only are the homemade versions better for you (less sugar, fat and preservatives), but they are actually much cheaper to make than to buy. The same thing goes for granola, fruit roll ups, sweet potato chips and more. Take some time to look up recipes of your favorites and see how much you can save!

As you can see, if you put a little time, thought and preparation into your food choices it can be easy to save some extra money! However, if all else fails, put things into perspective: Food is your form of medicine. By eating this way, you are preventing chronic disease and investing in lower healthcare costs. When looking at it in this light, remind yourself that it's okay to splurge every once in a while.

How to Talk to Your Loved Ones About This Change

As with any change in your life, your family and friends are going to ask questions. Most people are skeptical of any type of eating that is not centered around "conventional" or "convenient" foods. Just because we know better, doesn't mean that everyone else is in the loop. Don't worry! Thousands of people have been in your shoes before and have survived.

Each person has their own reason for adapting to an anti-inflammatory lifestyle. Is this diet going to help resolve health concerns such as arthritis, irritable bowel syndrome or celiac disease? Or maybe you want to prevent health problems that are associated with inflammation. Maybe you are just sick and tired of always being sick and tired. Tell your loved ones what your inspiration and motivation is!

Do some explaining. A large misconception about any type of diet is that you have to eliminate your favorite foods. While some foods are eliminated, they are also *substituted* with other foods so that you can still enjoy your favorite dishes. If someone is giving you a hard time because you aren't able to enjoy a plate of pancakes at breakfast, just remind them of how delicious our simple banana pancakes from days 1 and 5 are! Make sure to keep the ingredient list in mind. For example, let's compare Aunt Jemima's pancake mix to our recipe.

Aunt Jemima Original Pancake Mix: Enriched bleached flour (bleached wheat flour, niacin, reduced iron, thiamin, mononitrate, riboflavin, folic acid), sugar, leavening (sodium bicarbonate, sodium aluminum phosphate, monocalcium phosphate), salt, calcium carbonate

Simple Banana Pancakes: Coconut oil, banana, egg

I think you can agree that your body will thank you for choosing the banana pancakes!

Some people may simply be curious about your new habits. If someone is asking, enlighten them about some of your new food knowledge! Just keep in mind that not *everyone* is curious. Just like you don't appreciate friends and family criticizing your diet and forcing their food knowledge on you, you should not analyze their food or lecture them about their choices. Trust me, you don't want to be that friend. In the end, it is important to remember that this lifestyle change is about you, not about your friends or family.

References

Body Ecology, Inc. (2015). Retrieved from Stevia: www.stevia.net

Centers for Disease Control and Prevention. (2014, January 9). *Heart disease*. Retrieved from Centers for Disease Control and Prevention: http://www.cdc.gov/nchs/fastats/heart-disease.htm

Duyuff, R. L. (2012). *American Dietetic Association Complete Food & Nutrition Guide.* Hoboken, New Jersey: John Wiley & Sons, Inc.

Environmental Working Group. (2015). *Executive summary.* Retrieved from Environmental Working Group: www.ewg.org

Gedgaudas, N. T. (2009). *Primal body, primal mind.* Rochester, Vermont: Healing Arts Press.

Hoss, G. (2008, December 26). How It's Made. *12, 4.* Discovery Communications, LLC.

Lavallee, D. (2011, March 30). *URI scientist discovers 54 beneficial compounds in pure maple syrup.* Retrieved from The Univeristy of Rhode Island.

Liebman, B. (2015, June). Unscrambling eggs. *Nutrition Action Health Letter, 42*(5), 9-11.

Mercola, J. (2011, November 17). America's deadliest sweetener betrays millions, then hollywinks you with name change.

Morris, A., & Rossiter, M. (2011). *Anti-inflammation diet for dummies.* Indianapolis, Indiana: John Wiley & Sons, Inc.

National Honey Board. (2015). Retrieved from Honey: www.honey.com

Oh, J. (2012, April 30). *Average cost per inpatient day across 50 states in 2010.* Retrieved from Becker's Hospital Review: http://www.beckershospitalreview.com/lists/average-cost-per-inpatient-day-across-50-states-in-2010.html

Paleo Leap, LLC. (2015). Retrieved from Paleo Leap: www.paleoleap.com

Quinn, N. (2011, March 2). *The dreaded detox.* Retrieved from Paleo Plan: http://www.paleoplan.com/2011/03-02/the-dreaded-detox/

Runyon, J. (2014, February 6). *How to eat paleo on a budget.* Retrieved from Ultimate Paleo Guide.

Steve, D. E. (2011, October 14). *Green tea.* Retrieved from University of Maryland Medical Center: http://umm.edu/health/medical/altmed/herb/green-tea

Storage times for the refrigerator and freezer. (2015). Retrieved from FoodSafety.gov: http://www.foodsafety.gov/keep/charts/storagetimes.html

Team, T. P. (2015). *Beans and legumes: Are they paleo?* Retrieved from The Paleo Diet: http://thepaleodiet.com/beans-and-legumes-are-they-paleo/